Birthing Normally

a personal growth approach to childbirth

Gayle H. Peterson, MSSW, LCSW

with contributions by
Lewis E. Mehl, MD, PhD

preface by
Michel Odent, MD

photography by
Lyn Jones

Shadow & Light Publications
19861 Buck Ridge Rd · Grass Valley, CA

Acknowledgements

An abbreviated version of Chapter 11 originally appeared in the *Journal of Nurse-Midwifery*, April 1983 issue. It is reprinted here in revised form with the permission of the editor.

Portions of Chapter 13 were originally published in the *Birth Psychology Bulletin*, Volume 1, Number 1, for 1980 and in the *Journal of Nurse-Midwifery*, September, 1983 issue. We gratefully acknowledge the persmission of the editors of both of these journals to reprint any material which appeared therein.

An earlier version of the "Breastfeeding and Nutrition" Appendix appeared in an article by the authors in *Mothering*, Summer 1981. It is reprinted here in revised form with the permission of the editor.

Illustrations by Patricia Carvin
Photography by Lyn Jones
Production Coordination by Marian O'Brien
Cover Photography by Keith Whitaker
Back Photo by Linda Baziuk
Additional Contributors: Jo McRae, Ph.D.; Laura Grimes, M.A., M.D.; Lyn Jones, Pam England, C.N.M.

Library of Congress Catalog Number: 83-062343

To Sorrel Madrona,
and Yarrow Madrona,
for their beauty and inspiration to my work.

Contents

Preface
to the Second Edition

We must thank Gayle Peterson for developing a holistic model for childbirth in a time when it is most needed. In the field of traditional obstetrics to observe is often to disturb. Professionals have been too ready to use pharmacological and surgical intervention where emotional understanding was important. It is as if the modern professional is unaware that childbirth is a body and mind process.

A woman cannot be her freest to give birth if she is not culturally and personally permitted to express and integrate the emotional work of pregnancy and labor. The dynamics of the hormonal balance and equilibrium for labor can more easily flow if a mother has the freedom to express herself and to position herself in a setting of her liking. However, the most significant assistance that can be given a woman in birth is that assistance which will help her to resolve fears and anxieties. Each woman is uniquely individual, and our assistance as professionals must then vary in its nature to match the woman. We cannot approach every woman in the same manner and expect to have the same results. Gayle Peterson has understood the beauty of the individual woman at work to give birth.

Birth is not logical. It cannot be reduced to physiological analysis any more than the miracle of fetal development can be reduced to its description. *Birthing Normally* explores the crucial link between physiology and emotional experience. What has been thought of as instinct or intuitive knowledge are those feelings which interact with the hypothalamic limbic system for birth. Gayle's personal growth approach to childbirth makes sense of emotions, personal experience, and intuition as crucial aspects of a holistic model.

In a world where femininity and passivity are commonly associated, Gayle poses fundamental questions about attitudes of passivity and activity in labor and birth. Gayle Peterson is not only a psychotherapist. She is also a woman and mother. It is my belief that we must listen to mothers. They have a specific knowledge and understanding of life.

In a time when our planet is in danger for life itself, many people criticize male domination and control in every aspect of human existence, including childbirth. It may be that the first stage in an effective global revolution for peace will be when male doctors accept progressively to retire from obstetrics and return childbirth to women.

Birthing Normally reflects a woman's interior knowledge of birth as her most powerful resource for labor. In the predominantly male-oriented field of obstetrics, Gayle returns women to themselves for birth.

Michel Odent, M.D.
Pithiviers, France
September 1983

Introduction

THIS SECOND EDITION of *Birthing Normally* has been prompted in part by questions from readers — childbirth educators, midwives, physicians, nurses, pregnant women, and others. I owe further clarity of thought on birthing to the sharing and generosity of many people, including the critics of the holistic model for birth.

To begin, the definition of "normalcy" in birth has given rise to a surprising level of controversy, resulting from a confusion as to the reference point for normal. Is normal birth that which is socially "usual," and if so, are not Cesarean births (or other complications) usual and therefore "normal" in our society? From a social definition and use of the word "normal" as the "norm" (the "typical," "usual" or "average") naturally this would appear to be true. However it is not in a social context, but a biological context that the definition of "normal" birth is presented within these pages. Normal in a biological or physiological sense does not presume a social judgment, but is rather a purely functional term in biomedical usage. In medical charts and at medical conferences, the terms "unremarkable, N.S.V.D." (normal, spontaneous, vaginal delivery), and "normal" are used interchangeably.

My intent in using the biological "normal" is to keep biological normalcy in birth alive in the medical field as well as in our general society. The definition of normal birth in medical terms simply means the natural resolution of labor which does not require medical intervention and in which neither the life of the mother or child is threatened or compromised without such intervention. The fact of increased complication in birth in present society should not obscure our understanding of the normal process. We must not lose sight of normalcy in the face of our recent need for increased technological support in birth. But what contributes to this rise in complications?

Women are struggling, as are the men of our culture, in times of changing values which affect family cohesion and durability. The age of the nuclear family reached its peak and decline in the 1950's. A mother's rebellion from the powerless isolation of suburbia continues to reverberate throughout the 20th century. The fact that children and motherhood are naturally and biologically a part of womanhood inevitably renders childbearing susceptible to an increasing degree of unsettlement as women struggle for identity in economic as well as emotional terms. There is no question as to the absolute necessity for these changes, yet pregnancy and childbirth will be more conflicted for the average woman until the whole of society has adopted and adjusted to support the changing identity of women in the second half of our century. In a more general sense, the women's movement has indeed catalyzed needed changes for men and children as well. But as a culture we are only beginning to assimilate these changes.

The integration of mothering as a part of womanhood is not an easy task when women's socioeconomic equality may be riddled with challenge at best and oppression at worst[1].

Pregnancy has always been a time of stress, the natural and healthy stress of transformation to motherhood. Pregnancy, labor, and birth have always served as nature's bridge to mothering. It is a natural state of self-reflection and a time when a slight increase in anxiety may be generated and useful to fuel the psychological integration needed in becoming a mother.

The psychological task of pregnancy has been identified as the work of integrating the psyche to include the emotional construct of mothering[2]. Is it any surprise that complications in labor and birth increase with the difficulty of this task?

Society has been reduced to the smallest biological unit possible in childbearing — the single parent and child family. Never before has this smallest of family units been so prevalent. The fact that more women are choosing single motherhood than ever before, in a time when procreation is a choice, reflects the obvious increase in the stress of the role and identity of mother in our culture within a larger family context. Though by no means attaining a majority, there has been an increase in women choosing single motherhood over traditional shared parenthood. Some women report the stress of both relationship and mothering as overwhelming and markedly prefer to adapt to the adjustments of motherhood on their own[3]. In the course of history, single motherhood has never before emerged as a viable alternative. The fact that it is being chosen as such echoes the stress that has enveloped women as we quest for change on a societal and cultural level. The changing times of our society are a needed and creative stress born of the energy and potential for personal and cultural evolution. But our times are not without reflection upon the perinatal period, a period which already stimulates a natural increase of anxiety for integration of motherhood.

Our society is in flux, and is not yet supporting the woman of our times sufficiently in the mothering role. Yet women will continue to birth — to bring forth the needed children of humanity. The human race cannot wait for society to change in order to procreate with greater ease. As women, we are members of our society and will naturally strive to integrate the role of mother on an individual level. Our belief in motherhood is the beauty of our striving, and represents the lifespring of human existence today. However, the rise in obstetrical technology and intervention has confused the definition of "normal" birth. Confusion has occurred as a result of two very divergent but interdependent phenomena: the very real rise in need for technological support in birth in a transitional society, and the very real rise in complications resulting directly from *unnecessary* and/or *dehumanized* obstetrical intervention.

In response to distress the medical model has responded with more technological intervention. In a model in which bodies are viewed as machines, naturally intervention is aimed soley at the *mechanical* manipulation for resolving points of cumulative stress that may peak in the full force of a woman's labor. The medical model offers women the only support it knows — mechanical resolution. Medical intervention has served not only necessarily for physical manipulation of outcome, but in some cases unnecessarily for socialization to the cultural norm of "good patient." Physicians, in some cases, perform Cesareans as a means of quick relief from the normal pain of labor when the woman in labor does not "deal well" with the pain (i.e. in our culture, quietly and without complaining). An increase in technology beyond that already necessary in stressful times has resulted in a backlash of angry women who feel cheated of the opportunity for a normal birth[4]. Women have reclaimed their rights to nature, to their bodies in a manner necessary for society to remain alive and healthy. Consumer support groups have had effective and dramatic impact on obstetrical practice, as well as choices in alternative childbirth[5]. Women continue to be in the midst of reclaiming their rights to birth. Yet, times remain transitional in the 20th century, and having alternatives in childbirth available may not ensure a woman an easy transition into motherhood or an uncomplicated birth. Support of both a technological, in some circumstances, *and* an emotional nature, are needed. The need for increasing awareness of counseling as a natural part of prenatal care cries out to us. Availability of counseling services to support a woman's integration of mothering in a transitional society must be given if we are to use other than medical technology to reduce risk and to mitigate the stresses of the average modern woman entering motherhood.

How do we support women through the emotional integrative work of pregnancy without "blaming" ourselves or the pregnant woman for birthing outcome? What part of ourselves creates the potential to "blame" in order to recognize the impact of psychoemotional variables in the birthing process? Perhaps a social value judgement on "normal" delivery outcome is not necessary, but merely a by-product of a competitive society. The competitive society places judgement on "performance" in all areas of our lives, invading even the privacy of our most intimate experience — birth and sexuality.

It is exactly this dehumanizing principle of competition that women are struggling with as they enter the formerly male world of economics and career. As women and men in a changing world, we have already accepted the work for change in the last two generations and there is no turning back. We must travel through the labor of value reconstruction before we give birth to a new order. As women have entered the economical world, the economic values have entered woman's world of birth and procreation.

Perhaps it is the belief in competition, the erroneous interpretation of Darwin's theory of "survival of the fittest" which gives birth to the intention to blame a woman or a society for birthing outcome[6]. And it is blame itself that tightens and restricts our capacities to help ourselves and others.

Perhaps a bridging of the worlds of the health care system and consumer advocacy is possible through recognition of a broader cultural revolution and its impact on all of us. Compassion for ourselves as we bring about change — liberation from old values, understanding our potential for human joy, love, and creativity can eventually stabilize and secure the emotional identities of all of us who share the world at any given point in time. A society which places value on cooperation rather than competition will be more capable of supporting its members, including women bringing forth life to continue that society.

Birthing Normally addresses the need to keep sight of our biological definition of "normal." It does not serve women to be dissuaded from the biological "norm" in the name of unnecessary obstetrical technology. A 50% Cesarean rate should not replace a social normative for a biological definition of the normal[7]. For, if we are to stray too far, how will we return to that which is natural? How will our daughters return to a belief in their bodies to give birth? Nature may reflect a temporary stress of our times, however we must be clear in our knowledge of what is defined as "normal" biologically, so that the *average* woman now and eventually can return to biologically normal birth.

There is no success, no failure in birthing outcome within a holistic model. Blame becomes an anachronism. A truly holistic perspective is far *wider* than the traditional cause and effect, linear thinking of our times, on which traditional medical care as well as traditional psychology are based. Our minds need to broaden to express our heart's capabilities. Full discussion of holistic principles for birth can be found in *Holistic Prenatal Care* which describes and illustrates the philosophy of "Holism" in depth. *Holistic Prenatal Care* can serve as a reference for those who are left with questions that go beyond the pages of this second edition.

Birthing Normally is about the individual and creative way women adapt to the labor process, and about the natural and healthy stress a woman deals with in pregnancy as she adjusts to her baby to come. It is also about a woman's inevitable transformation as she hibernates that aspect of herself that will become mother. And it is about a journey, called labor, that delivers mother and child into each others' arms.

REFERENCES

1. Cooperstack, Ruth, "Psychotropic Drug Use Among Women," *Canadian Medical Association Journal,* 115:760–763, 1976; Stephenson, S. "The Impact of the Women's Movement: Implications for Child Development, Mental Health and Family Policy," *Canada's Mental Health Supplement,* 26(1), 10–13, 1978; Brown, G. W. and Harris, T., *Social Origins of Depression: A Study of Psychiatric Disorders in Women,* New York, Free Press, 1978; "Women and Health" Roundtable Report, Vol. II, No. 7, August, 1978.

2. See Chapter 2 of *Holistic Prenatal Care* for a more thorough discussion of pregnancy as a developmental task for families. Mindbody Press, Berkeley, in press.

3. The Finer Report on One-Parent Families (Report of the Committee on One-Parent Families. Cmnd. 5629. H.M. Stationery Office. Pounds 5.60 (2 volumes)) has estimated that there were 620,000 one-parent families in Britain in 1971 (with a total of 1,080,000 children). Ninety thousand (15%) of this substantial percentage of British families were unmarried mothers. At least 10% of all American families are single parent families, and it is estimated that as many as one out of five children live in a single parent family (Anstett, R.E., Poole, S.R.,and Morrison, J. The Single Parent Family. *The Journal of Family Practice,* 14(3):581–586, 1982). In cities such as Berkeley, California, estimates are as high as 50% single parent families (personal communication, Berkeley City Health Department, 1983).

4. Cohen, N. W. and Estner, L. J. *Silent Knife: Cesarean Prevention and Vaginal Birth After Cesarean,* Massachusetts, Bergin and Garvey Publishers, Inc., 1983.

5. NAPSAC, ICEA, C/SEC, CPM, etc.

6. The insights of systems biology have made clear the reality of cooperation in nature rather than competition and survival of the fittest as Darwin perceived. For further discussion of this topic, see Chapter 3 of *Holistic Prenatal Care.*

7. Cohen and Estner, *Silent Knife.*

Section I

Beliefs, Attitudes and Birthing

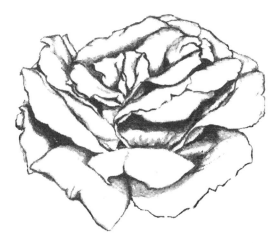

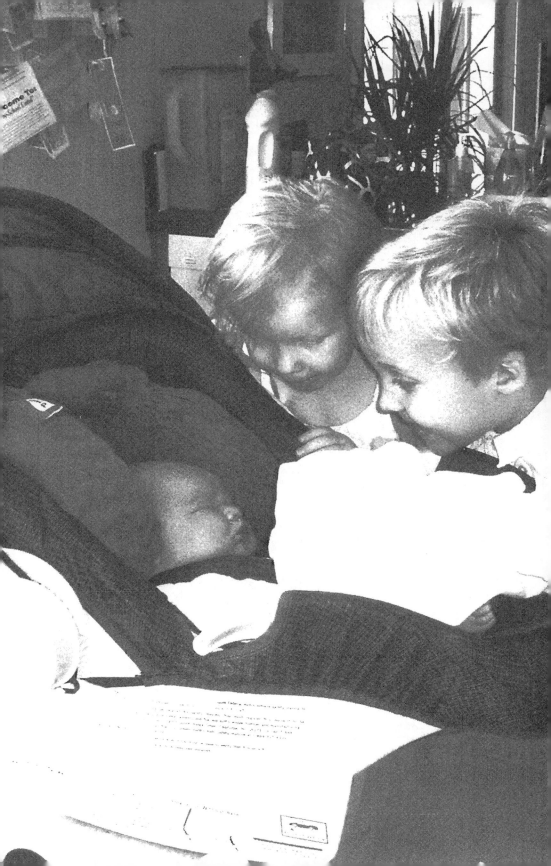

Chapter One

The Holistic Approach

As an increasing number of women are choosing to birth naturally and consciously, our society is experiencing a new kind of woman. A woman who prepares herself to grow during pregnancy (both psychologically and physically) is able to make the most of the creative and transformative nature of pregnancy, birth and motherhood. Current research has documented definite gains in self-confidence, and in psychological strength for women who have actively participated in the childbirth process.[1] Women who perceived themselves to be active, conscious participants in the birth process felt positively about their childbirth experience, and reported gains in self-confidence and self-esteem.[2] These were women able, with the help and support of friends, spouses, childbirth classes and supportive professionals, to approach birth in such a manner as to gain insight into themselves and their own psychological process.

As a woman lives, so shall she give birth, so shall she die; in like manner and style to her own individual approach to life. This is a basic assumption on which I build my theory of childbirth preparation. But life is not set. Changes occur. Times of change are often tumultuous, stressful, and often charged with emotional upset and transformation. Our most creative inspirations are born of a changed perspective which follows from a time of emotional upheaval, a period of creative stress.

Birth is a stress. Hopefully, it does not become *dis*tress. It is stressful for both newborn and mother. Birth is a natural stress which massages the baby from the womb outwards through a series of contractions of the uterine muscle, strong enough to push a baby outwards into the world. Such contractions stimulate a baby for breathing at birth. As the baby moves down the vagina its whole body is massaged and stimulated for breathing. This preparation for life is both healthy and realistic. The average length of 2nd stage (after cervix is fully dilated and baby descends down the vagina) in mothers of first babies has been 1½ hours, providing the birth is a natural one with no interventions necessary. During the 1½ hour period the baby moves forward during a contraction, then slips backwards a bit in between contractions, then surges forward again on the next contraction. In this manner the newborn dives its way out totally stimulated and massaged; this back and forth, and back and forth again journey helps the baby get rid of fluid and mucous from its lungs, as the pressure squeezes, stimulates and stresses the baby, just enough to make the necessary transition from womb to the outside world. Babies that experience an average second stage of 1-1½ hours generally come out very pink from the start, and begin breathing without any suctioning of mucous from the nose or mouth. Their cry begins after the breathing pattern has already been established and the cry is often not a very long, drawn out cry. Babies born with less stimulation in the second stage (many subsequent pregnancies) generally tend to appear a bit more bluish with the cry loud and lusty, marking the first breath with a start. Generally such crying serves to stimulate the baby's lungs and circulatory system, creating the stress needed for a healthy beginning. This particular creation of a healthy state of stress is a natural body mechanism in the newborn needed to complete the transition from womb to outside world.

Contrary to the belief that birth is traumatic, my experience with women birthing their babies has led me to a view of birth as a healthy stress. This stress seems necessary in order to orient the baby to life. The newborn's emergence into the world needs to be validated as a positive life change. That a baby is ready to make this change, if all is normal, is evidenced by the journey itself. Further clinging to the womb-like environment beyond the 9 month term would generate a life-threatening situation. By the time a baby has journeyed from the womb to the outside world, physiological changes have occurred which make it most ready for the mother's arms and breast; there is the point of destination.

As labor and birth is a time of creative stress for the mother as well as newborn, how a woman reacts to stress will be apparent in the labor process. A woman who has developed a style during her lifetime of being able to meet and handle stress without creating *dis*tress for herself, will be less likely to create blocks for herself in labor. Acceptance is the first step forward in the labor process.

Acceptance of pain, of the work presented by the foreseen task of actively giving birth, of journeying with the baby towards birth, smoothes the way for a progressive, natural labor and birth.

One of the most important duties a childbirth professional has is to present to women (and men) a realistic picture of birth. Realistic in terms of the body energy involved in the birth process. To protect a woman from the concept of pain in childbirth is to leave her without preparation for coping. Women who find themselves truly overwhelmed by the pain of birth, unable or unprepared to endure and transform the stress of labor to creative fulfillment (birth), are left with one of two choices: to flee from consciousness of the pain through drugs, or to react to their labor by developing a state of distress which is mirrored commonly, psychophysiologically, in uterine inertia, fetal distress, or other physical interpretations of stress. Physical complications can be natural developments of a state of emotional distress, as experienced by a woman either unprepared in life and/or childbirth classes for the reality of labor and birth.

Many childbirth professionals neglect to present childbirth realistically, especially to the primigravida. Hard work, discomfort, and other euphemisms do not prepare women who have never given birth before, for honest to goodness pain. Tapes of women in labor are often avoided or carefully chosen and edited so as not to frighten these new mothers-to-be. "Why talk about pain," one might ask, "everyone knows there's pain in birth, but we're trying to reframe it positively." This is the first mistake—to not deal with the issue of pain in depth, is to not address the source of much of the fear and struggle for "control." It is true that demystification of the physical process itself does help to alleviate fear, but the question of how to accept and work with pain towards the birth transformation itself is ignored. So, many women who planned to give birth naturally are without resources to deal with and make sense of the pain they find themselves experiencing. Perhaps they are "bad" or "mad" to be in such pain. Pain has been associated with suffering and punishment in our society and negatively viewed as "the lot of women" by many religions.

Pain remains the lot of the human race as we resist change, resist psychological growth necessary to free oneself to work towards fulfillment. Pain is an integral part of the life process, too. Virus and bacteria precipitate stress, pain and healing, in the process stimulating the development of our bodies to be strong, healthy, and sufficiently resistant. Psychological pain and stress endured during crises is often the way of transformation to new patterns of thinking and behavior. Psychological pain, when it is not transformed or assimilated into growth patterns, can lead to increased distress, to dissociative processes with resultant psychosis, depression or violence. Pain in childbirth, when it is not befriended and assimilated into a psychophysiologically integrated labor pattern, also increases as pain is perceived as overwhelming, dissociation occurs in the form of necessitated intervention. Resistance to pain in labor can become a source of physical complication. Since many women attempting to birth naturally would feel themselves to have failed, had they asked for medication, the more accepted pattern of coping is the development of a physical complication (such as uterine inertia), the body's way of saying, "Stop, I can't cope with this." This is truly a state of real distress, and compassion and support as psychological interventions serve sometimes to increase a woman's resources for coping. This real state of *dis*tress due to the unpreparedness of a woman for the realistic stress of labor and birth, is indeed a crisis situation and needs to be treated as such for the physical safety of both mother and child.

How a woman gives birth has been found to influence her confidence and ability to mother.[3] The more consciously and actively she gives birth, the greater is her confidence in her ability to mother, and long-term gains in self-esteem and self-confidence result.

The theory of childbirth preparation as it unfolds in the following pages is one in which the objectives that will be outlined are emphasized as a means of achieving the following goal: a state of psychophysiological integration which increases a woman's resources to deal with and transform stress of labor into creative fulfillment of birth. The creative fulfillment in this context is the natural childbirth the woman desires.

Childbirth classes based on this theory of psychophysiological integration have long-reaching effects into the life of the pregnant woman. A woman is helped towards preparation which increases her ability to handle stress. Childbirth preparation becomes preparation for life challenges and continued personal growth in the future. The ability to transform problems and conflicts into challenges is developed. The appropriate amount of stress (just as for the baby's stimulation for breathing) is needed, accepted, and harnessed as mobilization for attainment of the natural outcome or solution. The solution is more than the absence of the problem. It is a new development in terms of personal, psychological growth which enables a person to rise to a new definition of self. In childbirth the outcome takes the physical form of a baby. The new definition of self includes motherhood and a new relationship with the world. When the challenge defined is that of childbirth, definition of self needs to include a psychological readiness which results in confidence, endurance and yielding to the labor process.

Childbirth education focused on the development of resources to handle stress in labor has far reaching implications for other life processes. Other outcomes requiring a new definition of self, such as a new job, a new recognition of ability, can likewise become challenges which are approached more easily as inner resources of confidence, strength, and self-esteem have already been developed in the context of childbirth.

Some women require more preparation than others prior to childbirth. Much depends on the woman's present resources in terms of meeting stress: how she handles herself in the world and to what extent she takes control of her own life; whether she makes decisions passively or actively. In short, what I want to find out about each woman is her view of the world and her role in it. To achieve this understanding, I set up an interview with the woman or couple in order to plan or encourage preparing for the birth, as well as explore life changes involved in parenting. As a couple approaches the planning for birth and parenting, the individual world view is apparent within the context of the process. The couple's system, and role of each in relation to the other, also unfolds as information regarding passivity, activity and ability to communicate with one another is inherent within the birth planning. If this interview is done before classes begin, the childbirth professional is better able to know a woman's individual need for help in developing her own psychological resources. Individual work outside of the class environment might also be indicated. Confrontation of reality and fears can be a great catalyst in moving women towards themselves to look for the strength they need. More effective learning situations can be arranged when the childbirth educator knows the world view of each of her clients. In this way she can better assess the development of inner resources needed for childbirth. This kind of assessment can also be done within the context of early pregnancy classes, if they are small in number. Issues of fear, pain, and parental coping can be focused on as early as the first trimester, before women are actually ready to "prepare" for the birth itself.

I have designed childbirth classes for implementation in Holistic Prenatal Care which includes a course consisting of seven classes. Two classes take place early in the pregnancy, ideally between 2-4 months. Five later classes are consecutive and focused primarily on the birth, ideally ending approximately three weeks prior to birth. Within a holistic framework staff members provide classes as a part of prenatal care. Within such a holistic approach, the classes need not include extensive information on diet, complications of pregnancy or labor, or various hospital or medical policies, as these issues are handled in the course of the prenatal care. Classes can be limited exclusively to clients receiving prenatal care through the holistic program. In this way, health practitioners are assured of knowing clients as individuals, while simultaneously providing the possibility of group support for families travelling through pregnancy and birth together. Clients are self-selected for similar values concerning childbirth and their plans for their births, as they each choose to come to a holistic program which specializes in natural childbirth and holistic health practice. These kinds of programs are becoming increasingly developed throughout the United States and Canada, and are generally found in family practices. However, childbirth educators operating outside of a holistic model of prenatal care and childbirth education will no doubt need to lengthen the number of classes involved to approximately 10-12, for two reasons. The first reason is to insure the development of a relationship. Increased contact with the woman or couple is necessary, since outside of a holistic team approach, childbirth educators would rarely work as part of a health team involved in the prenatal care of their clients. Secondly, information concerning nutritional value in foods, complications of pregnancy and birth, and medical policy will differ for various women in the class to the extent that they are receiving prenatal care from a variety of doctors. Some doctors or midwives may include such information during prenatal examinations, and some will not. It will become necessary to make time during classes for these issues as needed.

Even without the ability to work inside of the holistic model however, childbirth educators can work to increase effectiveness of their classes by creating classes made up of a more homogenous group of people, so that issues addressed are equally relevant for all members of a class. Meeting clients to discuss their plans for birth prior to classes creates the opportunity to tailor the class to those people in it. By insuring optimal groups compatibility and cohesion, an atmosphere conducive to stimulation of personal growth is achieved. For example, a class made up of single mothers-to-be, or a class whose members are obtaining prenatal care from the same source, will create less necessity for repetition and specific issues addressed are more likely to be of equal concern and value to all members of such a class. In addition, a group support system is more likely to develop which can greatly augment resources available to expectant parents. Nuclear families as well as single mothers often desperately need such support, but find it difficult if not impossible to conceive of where to find it. Within the classes, encouragement can be given for group support in the form of baby sitting co-ops, emotional sharing, and friendships when they occur.

Included in this approach is the encouragement for women experiencing difficulty before, during or after attending childbirth classes to work privately on a one-to-one basis. For some women this may become a commitment to brief or long term psychotherapy. The considerations of individual work with the client will be discussed further as the book unfolds.

The Psychophysiology of Birth

A woman's belief in her body strength or weakness, as applied to birth is reflected in body language. Body posture and gestures bespeak the extent of a woman's comfort in her body and the space she occupies in the world. Daily integration of some kind of physical exercise is in general a healthy sign of respect and enjoyment of the body. Encouragement of daily exercise early in pregnancy stimulates awareness of the body and facilitates the integration of the psychophysiological model presented here. Recent emphasis on parental-infant bonding has clearly documented the emotional[4] and spiritual aspects of birth.[5] This is important. However, much too often recently, I find women so enthralled by the spirituality of the birth process and meeting their new babies that they all but forget that birth is very much a body process, just as pregnancy is.

The extent to which a woman's life philosophy validates the body's existence makes it easier to get to the place of uninhibitedness so essential in giving birth naturally and consciously. At some point in labor, a woman must make the decision to yield to the bodily experience, while simultaneously maintaining a field of strength and activity. As such, the labor is easiest met with an active and participatory yielding to the body work involved. For a woman to trust her body, she needs to be familiar with it. Relaxation exercises facilitate such body familiarity by consciously focusing the mind on the body muscles.

Trust of the body, of the body's ability to give birth, can be emphasized and validated in the present with respect to the current pregnancy. As a woman is growing, creating a baby human inside her own body, she can be directed to become aware of what her body is doing. She is creating form and structure in the shape of the human anatomy. She is creating internal organs, and the total foundation of a physical human including nerve networks and the incredibly complex network of the human brain. She is creating a placenta filled with lakes of blood, carrying oxygen and nutrients through the umbilical cord into the baby's circulatory system, carrying waste products away from the baby through different blood vessels in the cord back to the placenta and out through the mother's body system. A woman can gain confidence for birth through awareness of her pregnancy.

In addition, it is important to relate the woman's body knowledge in pregnancy to the process of labor and birth. During a visualization of the birth process, which is done in the first class of the holistic series of late classes (and/or privately on an individual basis), women are encouraged to trust their bodies. I teach pregnant women that they each know on a body level such information as the sex of the baby, when the baby will be born, and when conception took place. Bodily information is available because the woman's body is not confused. She is not making a boy, if she is making a girl or vice versa. Her body carries out the plan of nature without confusion and without interruption (assuming a normal course of pregnancy). However, this is all taught indirectly in the visualization process. More will be said about the visualization process and the use of hypnotic suggestion for cervical dilation and birthing in Chapter IV.

As a woman births, she crosses the boundary between unconscious and automatic mothering to conscious deliberate mothering. By this I mean that a woman is *already mothering* on a biological level before her baby is born. During pregnancy she is nurturing, feeding, and totally caring for and creating the developing baby inside of her. She is working hard, but all on an unconscious, automatic level. It is only after her baby is born that she will have to be sure it is warm enough, has enough to eat, is held and diapered. Breastfeeding is all that remains of the automatic mothering, although many hormones prime the mother for emotional bonding to the baby. By drawing attention to the physical work involved in pregnancy, body knowledge is validated and a woman's trust in her own body process during labor, birth, and lactation is developed. Again, how this material is taught is crucial.

Motherhood has remained in our culture the relatively invisible work of women. So is pregnancy also not recognized as a time of work for the mother. Because the work truly is invisible and internal, the physical work of pregnancy is not validated in our society. Women who are pregnant and working are indeed performing two jobs and should be credited with such. Fatigue in pregnancy need not give a woman a sense of inadequacy in her body, or negativity about her ability to "perform" in the world, if she is conscious of the tremendous body energy she is using internally. Adequate physical exercise coupled with an awareness of the specific work of pregnancy can build, early in the pregnancy, the sense of strength and yielding which is necessary for birth. Pacing and adjusting physically to each trimester within the pregnancy serves to develop mind-body integration, emphasizing responsibility for the decision to create new life.

During a first interview and throughout early and late classes, it is important to create awareness of this body knowledge and work of pregnancy within the individual woman's family system. This will serve to enhance the woman's sense of worth and confidence through her relationship with her man and/or labor support person.

As a woman journeys through labor and delivery, she experiences the transition from unconscious to conscious mothering. As such, giving birth is a process very much affected by the integration or lack of integration between the mind (conscious mothering) and body (unconscious mothering).

Psychological crisis can play an important role in the interruption or eventual complication of the labor. As mentioned earlier, psychological stress in the form of inability to cope with labor and pain in labor is a real stress to which the body reacts, discharging metabolites at an increased rate.[6] This is the body's mechanism for attempting to neutralize the effects of stress on the body. Psychological stress can present itself due to innumerable causes. The originating causes may take various forms, resulting in an inability to cope with labor. Unrealistic or minimal education to the childbirth process as well as psychological conflict can precipitate stress for labor. Psychological stress can be created by such issues as fear of motherhood, alienation from the body, loss of a previous baby through adoption or death, disharmonious couple relationship, unsupportive home situation, and/or feelings of personal inadequacy.

Awareness of Individual Growth Styles

As a childbirth professional and psychotherapist, I define childbirth preparation as meeting a woman on her own grounds as revealed in her approach to life. Each of us grows, psychologically and spiritually in like style to our living. Our style of living is reflected in everything we do, in everything we are. It is my responsibility to become familiar with the personal style by which that woman lives, because it is that style by which she develops psychologically, emotionally, and spiritually. And it is that individually creative style that can be nurtured, validated, and catalyzed for change as it becomes necessary for growth.

As a childbirth professional it is also my responsibility to attempt to facilitate such growth in helping a woman to meet her own vision of how she desires to give birth. Pregnancy, birth, and parenting are times of enormous change and can be opportunities for creative psychological growth and awareness as identities of individuals and families are formed and re-formed. Women become mothers, men become fathers, daughters become sisters, sons become brothers, and so on. As a pregnant woman's body grows and grows and grows and becomes, the mind is also full with this potential. And this potential is enlivened so much the more through the mind-body connection.

A part of the individual woman's approach to life involves various birth-related beliefs which may augment or diminish a woman's resources for giving birth. These we will now look at in the next chapter.

REFERENCES

Chapter 1

1. Peterson, G. and Mehl, L. *The Effects of Childbirth on the Self-Esteem of Women.* Publication no. 24, Psychophysiological Associates, Berkeley, California, 1980.

2. Peterson, G. and Mehl, L. Some Determinants of Maternal Attachment. *American Journal of Psychiatry*, 135:10, Oct., 1978.

3. loc. cit.

4. Klaus, M. *Maternal Infant Bonding.* St. Louis, C. V. Mosby, 1976.

5. May, I. *Spiritual Midwifery* (Matthew & Rachel Sythe, eds.) Sommertown, TN, Book Publishing Co., 1977.

6. Selye, H. *General Theory of Stress in Health and Disease*, New York, Butterworth, 1976; and *Hormones and Resistance*, Zurich, Springer-Verlag Publishers, Vols. I and II, 1971.

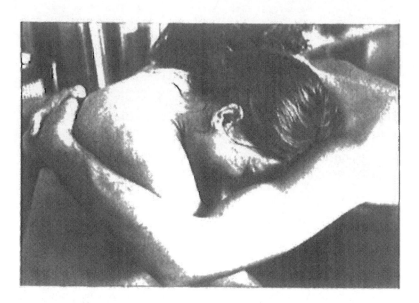

Chapter Two

Beliefs, Attitudes and Labor

THE PHYSICAL EFFECT of attitude on the body's resources has been documented in current research by the Simontons.[1] Attitudes of hopelessness, giving up, and victimization have been shown to be communicated physically through the limbic system. Changes in hormonal balance due to altered functioning of the hypothalamus affects the pituitary gland rendering an effect on the body of lowered resistance and stamina during these dejected emotional states. Psycho-emotional factors affect the immune system, lowering resistance, contributing to increased cancerous growth in cancer patients. We have found the psycho-emotional factors related to attitude to also affect the labor process. Predictability of delivery outcome is heightened by recognition of attitude and belief as producing profound effects in the body's resources.

Pregnancy, labor, and birth is a process existing within a greater life process of each individual woman. Psychological factors, existing within the woman herself, in addition to the interaction of environment and human relationship, are apparent in the labor. Recognizing psychological beliefs and attitudes affecting labor can render greater opportunity for uncomplicated labor and birth. Emotional strength, endurance and confidence are all qualities which enhance the possibility of success for any task undertaken, including childbirth. Facilitating the development of these inner resources is a goal of childbirth preparation as I view it from the holistic perspective of childbirth as an opportunity for personal growth.

Intervention of a psychological nature has not been tapped in the framework of the medical setting. It is not surprising that those birth attendants having the widest knowledge of psychological tools used in labor were initially lay midwives, who, unarmed by the usual drugs and tools of the medical profession, by necessity had to become aware of the psycho-emotional factors operating at any given moment in time. It is true, presently, however, that many of the new midwives who have joined the ranks because of the growing popularity of the popular profession, have ignored such precious knowledge, yearning instead to become ever more "medical" in their approach.

Regardless of the place of birth, psychological interventions during labor can be used. However, interventions of any kind, psychological or medical, presuppose a distress of some sort. Here it is the identity of the problem itself that defines the nature of intervention.

Such interventions of a psychological nature during labor will be discussed as an extension of the childbirth preparation classes in a later chapter. We as childbirth professionals want to help facilitate a natural childbirth without interventions of any kind, medical or psychological, to the extent that is possible. Preventive therapy in the form of childbirth classes which facilitate an inner development of a woman's own psycho-emotional resources to better meet, accept, and work with pain in labor can create less need for intervention of any kind. As a woman needs intervention of either a psychological or medical form, so does she have every right to such support, and should not have to create a physical drama (such as hemorrhage) for her cry for help to be heard. Physical complications are often precipitated by psycho-emotional stress which goes unrecognized until such stress is transformed into physical form. This is particularly true in the case of fetal distress. Metabolites produced by a fetus in an attempt to neutralize psycho-emotional stress experienced by the mother are dramatically apparent in the evidence of premature labors occurring at a heightened percentage during air raids and attacks during time of war.[2] Such effects of stress, however mild or severe, are traditionally addressed only as they are transformed into physical complications. This is the medical model. By including the psychological and emotional spheres of the pregnant woman as part of prenatal care, we are providing a model for preventive obstetrics. Childbirth education becomes an integral part of a holistic approach to prenatal care, as psychological development of inner resources is emphasized as a means of meeting and transforming psychological stress, before physical effects of such stress become problematic.

It is imperative that we also give support for making a responsible decision to give birth by teaching a woman that she can give birth and that only *she* can do it. No one else can push her baby out, except by intervention. Too often, childbirth classes lead women to believe they should be pampered throughout their labor. This sabotages a woman's source of strength. A woman within the mind-space of a baby herself finds it very difficult to birth her baby. Emotional support in the context of the reality of the experience better prepares a woman to give birth, have pain, and accept emotional support for such hard work. A woman treated with respect for her strength will believe in herself.

Particular birth-related beliefs can augment or diminish the impact of the overall resources a woman has present within her self-identity. Let us begin with a look at some major psychological issues and their possible effects on the labor process, as potential resources or complications for a natural childbirth.

Activity vs. Passivity

Labor is an active body function. The more active a woman is, both physically and in the form of decision making in her own life, the closer she is to familiarity with the labor process. The greater her passivity for decision making and physicality, the less prepared she is for the active work of labor. Likewise, the more self-reliant a woman is capable of being in her life, and the more independent, when *coupled with* the ability to also accept needed emotional support from others, the greater her ability to adapt and yield to her labor.

A woman who feels she is in active control of her life and in general takes responsibility for her actions and behavior in the world, finds herself able to take control of her labor experience. She feels "up to" it. It does not strike her as insurmountable. She is able to remain in the present, working with each contraction to bring her baby down through her body. She does not view herself as a victim. Birth feels powerful, contractions are viewed as a part of herself. She is at one with her body, for all the intensity of labor. Expression of pain is in part her union with her body accepting labor as the body experience it is, particularly in hard labor. The ability to view oneself as active in labor can be taught, and is a resource for the laboring woman.

The Ability to Be Uninhibited

As a woman births, she comes to a place of lack of inhibitions necessary to push her baby out of her womb and into her arms. The level of inhibitedness present in her life in general bespeaks how far a woman has to stray from her accepted inhibitions to this place of being uninhibited and open for birth. The more familiar she is with expressing herself through her body, the greater is her familiarity with such bodily freedom. Expression, such as singing, yelling, dancing, and sports are all active states and as such stimulate mental attitudes associated with self-reliance and activity in general. The ability to express oneself, and to become less inhibited about such expression during labor can also be taught and becomes a resource for the laboring woman. Feeling free to express herself in any way she might choose during labor facilitates deepening relaxation associated with the lack of inhibition.

Victimization

The extent to which a woman excuses her behavior as the result of being a victim, whether a victim of disease, circumstances, or finances, the more practiced she becomes at viewing herself as not responsible for events in her life. Labor becomes another event, one in which she can easily fall into the trap of passivity in the victim role. The pain of labor is viewed as external rather than as coming from her own body. She feels victimized by the process, by the pain involved, and becomes alienated, if not hostile to, her own body. In such a state of disharmony and conflict between mind and body, tension is increased and energy is often bound into such an intense clash of purpose as to result in a developing pattern of uterine inertia. Such inertia may be precipitated by a state of extreme fatigue and lack of confidence due to the inner war of victim, the woman vs. oppressor, the labor. As victim, she becomes alienated from the process, alienated from her body. It is not surprising that within such a view, a woman may feel the need to give up, or may spend vital energy needed for labor on an internal battle against her oppressor, which in this case is the labor process itself. Such an attitude is a drain on her inner resources and needs to be transformed into a positive image of strength and yielding which can be taught in classes and encouraged on an individual basis. Direct confrontation of the issue of pain in childbirth classes is essential in preventing possible victimization from occurring during labor.

Low Self-Esteem and Body Image

Women who identify strongly with the belief that they are weak or frail find it difficult to summon up the resources they do have for the work of a natural childbirth. A view of one's self in the world as strong physically and emotionally creates a higher level of self-esteem and confidence which becomes a resource for a woman in labor, and in mothering as well. To the extent that a woman views her body as healthy and resistant to malady and disease, the greater is her trust in her body and in herself. Trust in the body is an important stepping stone in achieving a state of psychophysiological integration which will enable a woman to develop self-confidence as a resource for giving birth.

Awareness of Fears, Conflicts and Concerns About Birth and Parenting

No matter how a woman relates to each issue presented here, a very important influence is her ability to see herself where she is. Awareness of a particular fear, conflict or concern is the first step towards resolution. The mere acknowledgement of fear and receiving support for such expression is a great tension reliever for the women I have worked with. To experience fear and to hide it from one's self is to create a double tension —one based in the fear and a second layer of tension rooted in the covering up of this fear from one's self and others. The result is free-floating anxiety without known cause, but influential in maintaining a constant level of persistent tension. This persistent anxiety and tension is the body's way of attempting to express the inner conflict, so that it can be recognized and dealt with. The variety of fears or conflicts involved in such an occurrence are as widely varied as the individuals themselves. Fears of inadequate body strength to fears of mothering and potential loss of a partner through parenthood are but a few examples.

Recognition of those at risk for inabiltiy to cope with labor can be made from a study of the woman's present approach to life. The manner in which a woman may handle labor is generally reflected in her ability to respond to her body actively with little inhibition, perceiving herself as both strong and powerful during the labor process. Integrating the concept of pain into her preparation for labor and birth reduces the possibility that victimization might predominate in the actual experience of labor.

Pregnancy is a developmental process and the psyche of a

woman develops in response to the increased momentum of the pregnancy. As the time of birth draws near, a woman is moving towards resolution of conflict, expression of any existing conflict, or a certain culmination of whatever life process is reflected for her in the microcosm of completion of the fetus.

Pregnancy is the shortest complete life cycle of human evolvement available for observation. Within the womb, a fetus develops and prepares for life outside. The fetus is made with all the body equipment necessary for breathing, but does not actually breathe until the moment of birth when a new life cycle begins. When a woman reaches her last month of pregnancy it becomes more apparent whether she is in fact ready to give birth. If she is not ready psychically, this will be revealed in her body carriage, her response to slides of birth, a feeling projected outward of not being finished or prepared. Most often it is in the form of anxiety of a free-floating sort. This is usually accompanied by a quietness, a restless agitation and air of denial. Stress becomes increasingly evident between the man and woman if this anxiety remains unnamed. Sometimes, the mere recognition of it will bring a woman to the point of resolution needed to open her to birth. As she realizes that she does not have to be without fear, she becomes more able to accept the inevitability of nature, rendering herself more yielding to the process.

A case example will serve to illustrate this point.

Lana was a 36 year-old woman expecting her first baby. She was somewhat worried about her age, since she had been warned of complications by her former doctor, since she was having her first child at age 36. She had chosen to come to a holistic health center (where I was employed as a Birth Counsellor) to prepare for a home birth, since she could not use the Alternative Birth Center due to her age (this age restriction has since been dropped by the hospital). Throughout pregnancy and childbirth classes, Lana remained tense and quiet. Her husband was quiet and withdrawn during classes as well. Communication observed between them during classes and prenatal exams was terse, with indirect eye contact. Both of them were becoming increasingly passive as Lana entered her last month of pregnancy. During her last 4 weeks of pregnancy, Lana's baby turned transverse and remained there for the next 2 prenatal visits. At 2 weeks before her due date, I called her and asked her to come over to talk about pregnancy, labor and breastfeeding. As we began discussing the coming birth, it became very clear that Lana was not confronting herself with the reality of her situation. She knew she would have to go into the hospital if her baby did not turn head down, however she was not confronting herself with the inevitability of Cesarean section should the baby not turn either head down or breech by the time labor ensued. As she became aware of the physical reality of her situation, Lana put both hands on her pregnant uterus and wondered aloud if she was not letting this baby turn head down due to her fear of labor and of becoming a mother. Lana went on to associate her fear directly to her behavior. She had been hiding her fear from herself. She wasn't quitting her work as she had planned and had secretly wished the baby would come early, before she had prepared things. She hadn't visited with her mother to decide whether or not she would like her presence at the birth. She had been behaving as if birth might not happen, yet wishing it would come early just to get it over with. This pointed towards an emotional attitude of non-participation in the birth process, brought on by unrecognized fears and anxieties. These anxieties increased as the time of birth drew near. She realized that she and Noel, her husband, had avoided the subject of the birth with one another, each feeling that they should not express anything negative about the birth or the coming baby. I encouraged Lana to feel her fear and supported her in being afraid. She resolved to quit working the next day, to visit with her mother, prepare her house, and talk with her husband about her fears and her right to express them. Lana became much calmer and much more relaxed in appearance as she became aware of her feelings and did not have to hide her fears from her husband, others and herself. Three days later, one and one-half weeks prior to delivery, Lana's baby turned head-down. Lana went on to deliver an 8 pound healthy baby girl at home after a 6 hour labor.

Lana had heard all of the class information, preparations and had catalogued it away for use after she had accepted the inevitability of labor and motherhood. The physical changes in her manner and body carriage after her confrontation of her fears were remarked on by 5 different people on the staff of the health center where she was receiving care.

Unresolved, unrecognized conflicts can be noticed in pregnancy and interventions can be initiated to help spur the development of the pregnancy to its final healthful stage of uncomplicated birth. Where existing conflict is not recognized or worked through either in pregnancy or labor itself, complications may show themselves in labor necessitating intervention of some kind.

The emphasis of the theory of childbirth preparation as a personal growth model is one in which conflict is recognized and addressed. Confrontation of the reality of labor and delivery can be a form of confrontation of an individual's resistance to growth and change. Labor and birth *is* growth and change; change for the fetus, the mother, the family unit. The change of assimilating a baby into a family is also a point of stress. Bonding to the baby immediately after birth is a healing phenomenon for that stress. Assimilation of the newborn into the family becomes easier as the commitment to parenthood is accepted. As a family can experience the creativity and wonder of birth, the emotional involvement in labor becomes that parental commitment which is born with the baby. Immediate acceptance of the baby becomes the boon for dealing with this extraordinary adjustment in the family. Acceptance of the baby into the family begins with education to the realities of the labor process itself and direct confrontation of such realities as necessary. Gentle and firm confrontation, as illustrated in this example, paved the way for Lana and Noel to fully experience and participate in the labor and birth process as originally planned, the result being an optimal bonding experience to their new baby. Adjustment to parenthood was easier as Lana in particular had opened herself to her fears prior to the birth, creating a conscious life transition. Lana's body did not have to express unvoiced psycho-emotional conflict in the form of physical tension and stress which could have caused complications in labor.

The interaction of mind and body becomes apparent. Psychological distress or conflict predisposes the body to a physical tension and stress which consumes available energy and resources, as well as interfering in the normal hormonal and neurochemical changes of any body process, such as childbirth. In addition, metabolites produced physically as a normal response to neutralize psychological stress in the body, cross the placental barrier. The fetus reacts by also producing metabolites in an attempt to neutralize the effects of stress on its body. [3] With this interaction of body and mind, it becomes easier to understand fetal distress within the context of mind-body integration, when both the psychological and physical state of the mother are given equal concern and attention. Such knowledge can be used preventively in prenatal care and classes by addressing such issues as the one mentioned in the case above.

Augmentative Beliefs for Labor

In addition to developing a set of resources for childbirth as discussed in the context of the above-mentioned psychological issues, there are innumerable beliefs or circumstances which can influence the labor process for the positive. The following is a list of three categories of beliefs and attitudes conducive to labor and birth. Identification of these attitudes or beliefs is essential for accurate assessment of resources for natural childbirth. It is of extreme importance to get to know the client individually in order to understand the weight of significance any of the above resources or the categories of birth-related beliefs might have in life.

For example, a woman may have low self-esteem and a negative attitude towards her body, yet be able to yield easily to birth because of a dominant tendency towards being uninhibited. She may follow her body through the process in a trusting manner once she has reached that point of lack of inhibition in herself. As a childbirth educator and/or attendent for such a woman, it would be extremely helpful to observe this tendency so that this established, natural resource could be facilitated early in the labor.

For such a woman, then, body image and self-esteem may not carry the weight of significance that the tendency towards uninhibitedness does and so are not necessarily influential in blocking the ability to give birth. However, development of self-image and self-esteem could only improve her resources to deal with labor as well as other life processes.

Each woman is infinitely creative in her existent resources and the interaction of learning and experience. This originality evident within the individual needs always be respected, and as such, the element of surprise is always a possibility. By refining our abilities to ascertain various resources and working towards their development, a greater spectrum of creative potentialities exist for working with women for facilitation of a normal, healthy delivery.

The greater knowledge we have of the woman and her family system, the greater is our ability as childbirth professionals and other health care workers to facilitate the natural healthy outcome desired.

1. Body Image

A strong sense of trust in the body can lend confidence to a woman's belief in herself to give birth. Familiarity with the body, through sports, dance, or other physical activity, creates a growing expression of physical strength, as well as a feeling that the body is accessible and therefore trustworthy in labor.

This includes a history of having respected the body as both a source of enjoyment and as an extension of experience. Fulfillment through the body in terms of challenges of an artistic nature (dance, gymnastics) and/or through the senses (sex, swimming) in which the *total* body is active, can be a pillar of confidence in labor. Bodily experience is not new or alien for such women. Labor is very much a bodily experience, in addition to being an emotional and spiritual one.

A woman's belief in her body, how she views her body image, can directly influence her ability to use her body to birth her baby, to push it out. Viewing her body as strong, capable, and "in shape" lends more confidence to her ability to labor and birth. Exercise is particularly important in pregnancy and should be encouraged for its psychological as well as physical benefits for labor.

2. Beliefs about Birth and Past Experience

The more that a woman grows up with a positive attitude about birth, the more relaxed and confident she is. Attitudes are learned emotionally. When attitudes are changed, they are changed through re-learning on an emotional level. Slides of labor and delivery, shown from a positive perspective, can reach a woman emotionally and help her to re-learn pregnancy, labor and birth as a positive experience. Such reawakening needs to occur from an emotional level, affecting a person profoundly enough to change a basic learned view of childbirth.

3. Beliefs about Womanhood

The more a woman's concept of womanhood includes both a belief in women as strong and capable, and validates the creative potential available to women in the form of creating life, the less conflicted are her feelings of identity. As her physical form changes, it becomes a strong and creative feeling of powerful potential as opposed to a weak or burdensome feeling of degradation or suffering. This concept of power and creation in pregnancy can be conveyed in childbirth classes and throughout holistic prenatal care.

Diminutive Beliefs for Labor

Diminutive beliefs are beliefs or attitudes which diminish a woman's overall resources for labor. The following four categories of beliefs and assumptions need to be recognized in relation to the weight of significance that each may carry for the individual woman. Each belief is discussed with attention to its effects as an attitude which predominates in the individual personality.

1. Body Image

As a woman dislikes her body, she becomes alienated from it. A disgust for her body functions may also accompany such dislike. Anything that reminds her that she has a body creates tension. Attention on the body is often of a negative kind. A history of illness tends to diminish respect and trust for the body. Such negative feelings and experiences connected with the body create a negative view of labor as it is a body function. The inability to adjust to the pregnancy may be apparent early, and can be dealt with as soon as it is identified.

2. Beliefs about Birth

Terrifying or dehumanizing tales of childbirth couched within a woman's childhood education and/or experience breeds fears ranging from humiliation to maternal death. Fear of humiliation due to the learned view of childbirth as a degrading experience, but one that a woman feels she "has to go through" to "get a baby" are damaging to the sense of confidence, power, and strength needed in labor. Intense fears of maternal and/or fetal death need to be identified and addressed as early as possible, while simultaneous exposure to a view of childbirth as healthy, normal, and powerful needs to be introduced. This kind of exposure can take place in early pregnancy classes.

3. Past Experience

This catagory refers to past experience of loss or grief associated with an earlier pregnancy, labor and birth. In particular, a previous experience of adopting a baby out tends toward significant conflict in labor, as the experience of labor takes the woman back to memories of that earlier time in her life when her body enacted a like process. When this process is associated with emotional trauma and loss, conflict is common. Mothers who have previously adopted out, or lost a baby through crib death, accident, or disease soon after birth, are often flooded with painful memories at the next labor and may require psychotherapeutic work to emotionally accept the present baby as a new and different being from the one formerly lost.

These women need in-depth work during pregnancy and labor to support and encourage any necessary grieving and the expression of anxiety, fear, or guilt. Such women often present special needs that are best dealt with on a highly individual basis outside of and in addition to childbirth classes.

The following case example illustrates how one woman was helped to accept the past loss of a baby to facilitate enjoyment and experience of the present pregnancy.

Jocelyn was a 24 year old woman with a history of three past abortions. She came to a holistic oriented health center for prenatal care in her 4th month of pregnancy, planning a natural childbirth. During prenatal visits, it was suggested to Jocelyn that she come to see me to talk about her past abortions which were troubling her greatly and causing her depression. She expressed guilt over the abortions and ridiculed herself continually for her previous inability to be ready for motherhood. She was extremely tense and fearful of her ability to carry her present pregnancy, and her right to be a mother. She was experiencing alienation from this present pregnancy as a result of guilt feelings about one abortion in particular which took place at 5 months gestation several years previously.

Jocelyn was guided through reliving the memory of her labor with that baby, of seeing her baby born and being able to look, touch, talk to, and say goodbye to the aborted baby. She had not been able to so much as look at her baby when the abortion was actually taking place. As it was 5 months gestation, Jocelyn had experienced labor and birth as a part of the abortion process, but had never been able to say goodbye or to explain her feelings to the baby she was losing. Jocelyn cried and talked to her baby, expressing grief that was long overdue. She grieved for her baby, for herself, and for her lost motherhood. She said good-bye to her baby, and during the next 2 weeks wrote a letter of farewell to the little lost being.

When Jocelyn finished her farewell letter she was greatly relaxed. Her depression had lifted, and she smiled and talked excitedly about the baby inside her. She was now happy to feel the baby's movements inside of her and expressed a feeling of closeness to the present fetus. No longer burdened by guilt, Jocelyn had relieved herself of the need for punishment. She had worked through the grief process and was now free to discover and enjoy the baby she was to give birth to in 5 months.

Through her grief process, Jocelyn had separated her past loss from her present pregnancy. With this work done, Jocelyn will face less chance of repercussions of unresolved guilt and anxieties surfacing during labor. She will also be free to bond to this present baby with lessened chances for the projection of guilt, punishment and resentment onto the new baby. Aside from complications in labor, such unresolved guilt could have kept her from knowing this baby for who he or she is, and from being the mother to this baby that she is now capable of being.*

An example of the resolution of a loss through adoption with the help of brief-term therapy is illustrated in the following case example.

Barbara was a 28 year old woman who was planning a home delivery. This was her second pregnancy. Ten years earlier she had given birth to a baby which was adopted out. During the initial interview (a routine birth counsellor interview included in the holistic prenatal program) Barbara was unable to recall any part of the past birth experience. She seemed afraid of remembering the past, and spoke to me about this pregnancy and birth as her first. This was her husband's first baby as well. It was suggested to Barbara at about 7 months of pregnancy, that she might benefit from coming to see me for relaxation training to help her during birth. It was also suggested by her midwife that the actual physical occurrence of labor and delivery could stimulate memory of the past birth experience, which she had suppressed, and that she might benefit from uncovering the past birth experience to see what it had been like for her.

Barbara came for therapy sessions 4 times in the next 6 weeks. Because of the imminence of the birth, this timing (7 months gestation) was a perfect stimulus for motivating Barbara to do the

---

*Jocelyn experienced a normal, natural childbirth after a 5 hour labor. She gave birth to a healthy 7 lb. baby girl.

work she needed to do. There is often less resistance to needed psychological work as a woman nears the last 2-3 months of pregnancy. Prior to the third trimester, women do not feel so much the reality of the pregnancy and the sense of immediacy that becomes increasingly dominant as the date of delivery nears. In this way timing can play an important role in lessening psychological resistance.

Barbara participated in a reliving of her birth 10 years ago, during her first session. In a relaxed state she was able to visualize and remember the labor, her feelings of shame and inadequacy, and her guilt about her son. As she worked through the experience, she was able to create change in her visualization, to give herself the right to hold and touch her baby, to say good-bye to her son. She had not been able to hold, look, and talk to her son when that birth had actually occurred. Visualizing her son, she was able to feel the loss she had so long denied herself, and her grief poured forth. She also became aware of her gift of life to him. She was able to move towards acceptance of her actions and resolution of a loss never acknowledged. In looking back, she not only uncovered pain, but also beauty and a sense of having given birth once before, which lent her confidence for this birth.

The second session, Barbara created a visualization of meeting with her now 10 year old son, of knowing him, and finding herself unafraid of the truth of her motherhood. Barbara had previously been tense and afraid of the possibility of ever being searched out by her son. After her second session she was not fearful of this possibility, but felt she might even welcome it, should it occur. During this time, she had accepted her past and so reclaimed a part of herself which she had denied for 10 years. As she reclaimed her past, she experienced the beauty and strength in the experience of her first birth which could act as a resource for the coming labor and delivery.

During her third session, Barbara's focus was on her present pregnancy, and a visualization of the birth experience as it could be for her this time. The completion of a labor with the birth of the present baby which she would now keep and mother was a fulfilling and exciting visualization experience for Barbara. She was free of psychological guilt. Distrust of her body's association to her first childbirth was no longer a burden for her.

Barbara came in a 4th time with her husband, who had been experiencing some performance anxiety around his role as "labor coach" to his wife. A deeper understanding of his own coming identity as a father lessened his anxiety about the birth, and further cemented their commitment to one another in relation to themselves and the family they were creating.

Barbara's first childbirth no longer remained a denied part of her, but could be remembered in the present as a source of strength and confidence at her having created life and given birth once before. Having accepted her loss and grieved the necessary separation from her first child, Barbara did not need to suppress guilt and unresolved emotional pain during her present childbirth. She was free to validate herself as a woman giving birth for the second time. She had given birth once before, 10 years ago, and her body could now guide her present child into her arms. The present baby she could now accept as a new individual who was hers to mother.

Through 4 counselling sessions during the last trimester of pregnancy, Barbara was able to transform past shame and failure into a present resource for birth and mothering. Anxiety about a possible meeting of her first child no longer plagued her as she became free to be the person she was. She gave birth naturally to an 8½ lb. baby boy at home, after 4 hours of active labor.

4. *Negative Identity As A Woman*

If a woman's definition of womanhood is weak, fragile, or passive, or in contrast, if identity as a female is denied in an effort to deny acculturation of women as weak and inferior, she suffers an identity crisis in pregnancy which, if not resolved, can be brought to a crisis situation in labor. If a woman views herself as weak, she does not create the image of herself necessary to give birth, for labor is hard work. If a woman views womanhood as strong, but only as long as womanhood does not include childbearing, she is equally in conflict and is also unable to include labor and birth in her self-image.

In an effort to redefine our identity, we as women have fought to become liberated, to be "equal to men". In some extreme circles, the fervor of "equality" has ironically become an unrecognized belief in male supremacy, resulting in the denial of the physical functions of pregnancy and birth in the name of the women's liberation movement. Paradoxically, test tube babies and the complete separation of pregnancy and birth from the body becomes the goal of what I believe is a reactionary response to male domination. A revolutionary response is one currently underway whereby women deny none of their rights to their own bodies and determine instead to take full control of the energy coming through them in pregnancy and birth as well as any other part of their life. As we as women fully participate in and take responsibility for giving birth as we choose, we are aware of our own power and strength in doing so. It is a power and strength unique to women alone, and without reference of experience for men. Men can be supportive and lend emotional strength and endurance to their partners, but they cannot give birth or ever experience the power of birth that a woman can. Out of this evidence comes the unrecognized birth envy. Though not given full recognition, birth envy is the silent sister of the much proclaimed penis envy postulate put forward by Freud.[4] Perhaps it is even the reason for the development of the penis envy assumption.

If a woman decides to have a baby, but has a hard time validating her strength without invalidating her pregnancy, or vice versa, she becomes caught in an identity crisis involving pregnancy, birth and motherhood. To become resolved, she needs to move towards relearning her concept of womanhood. She needs to examine the qualities she has attached to pregnancy in the past and become able to validate her pregnancy as a part of womanhood as she learns to view both womanhood and pregnancy as strong, creative, powerful concepts. I have too often witnessed a self-identified feminist denying her own validation in pregnancy; viewing herself as degraded, humiliated, and burdened and denying these feelings at the same time. Such a woman has not totally relearned her concept of womanhood, and she robs herself of a natural born right, her right to enjoy the power of creativity in full life form. Here again, special and individual attention needs to be given to such a woman.

The following case example illustrates this negative identity crisis and how it was resolved through recognition of these beliefs and attitudes during pregnancy, labor and birth.

Heather was a single woman, pregnant with her first child, who had recently moved to the Bay Area from Florida. She began coming to me for pregnancy counseling in her 5th month of pregnancy. She was planning a natural childbirth and was referred to me by her doctor to resolve her ambivalence about this pregnancy, ambivalence about motherhood, and intense anxiety about becoming a single parent. Heather felt used by her boyfriend and was struggling through her own negative identity as a woman and mother-to-be.

Heather had decided to ignore the pregnancy and avoid the discomfort of an abortion until she was too far along to obtain one. At that time, she moved to the Bay Area to avoid facing her intense personal identity crisis in the nonsupportive atmosphere of criticism from her family and friends. She had decided she would keep the pregnancy out of a desire to keep something that belonged to her, rather than adopting out. She instinctively felt a need to experience her childbirth in an active manner. Through her intuitive nature, Heather had guided herself towards a path of active participation in the birth process and of fulfillment in the female processes of pregnancy, birth and mothering. During her pregnancy she was faced with an internal war in which the battleground was her core identity as a woman. Many beliefs had to be changed before she would be able to experience fulfillment of a journey on which she had embarked . . . that of pregnancy, birth and motherhood.

She struggled with her own fears of being "like her mother" and had initially denied herself the right to any process which reminded her of her mother. She had wanted to define herself as "unlike" her mother; as a feminist, as a woman of strength and character. She found herself somewhat humiliated by her pregnant form, which reminded her of her mother's pregnancies. She had felt oppressed by her pregnancy, thereby denying herself the enjoyment of a process she had a biological right to as a woman. Her identity as a feminist woman did not include pregnancy, birth and mothering. Because of this, she found herself shamed by her female body, and at odds with her unborn child.

Intense psychotherapy in the second and third trimesters stimulated Heather towards an acceptance of her womanhood. Heather became accepting of her pregnancy as a valid aspect of her womanhood. She was encouraged to draw symbols of pregnancy and birth. Art therapy acted as a catalyst for transformation of shame of her female pregnant body to validation of beauty and power in her ever more pregnant feminine form. She moved towards yielding to her femininity in the biological nature of pregnancy and birth. As she did so, she also yielded to her unborn child. By the end of her eighth month of pregnancy, Heather had been able to accept the idea of having a boy child, should the baby be male. Previously, she had been unwilling to accept the possibility of carrying within her womb a male form. By the end of her pregnancy, Heather had redefined her identity as woman to include the right to pregnancy, birth, and motherhood as a valid choice. She found that she did not have to give up her strength and power in her re-definition.

Heather gave birth naturally, after a 6 hour labor, to a 7 lb. baby girl. Psychotherapeutic manipulation of the environment in terms of people present in the birth room was all that was necessary to resolve uterine inertia (cessation of contractions) in second stage. Uterine inertia, particularly in second stage, has occurred in the great majority of cases in my experience when women express significant ambivalence about the unborn child after the fifth month of pregnancy.

During the five months of psychotherapy, Heather's growth process had shown itself: she would gain insight into her conflict and then resist resolution for a period of time in which she would become increasingly adamant about her inability to resolve an issue. She would then begin talking herself into distress over her exhaustion at her effort, becoming increasingly ineffective until a point where she retreated into herself for responsibility for the conflict. At this point she was able to move towards resolution, as she accepted personal responsibility. Heather's growth process in labor remained the same. She denied early contractions as an extremely painful backache, which kept her awake in the night. She did not associate the pain to labor, even though the pain was severe as her baby was posterior. This was similar to her denial of her early months of pregnancy. When Heather arrived at the alternative birth center at the hospital, she was 7 centimeters dilated. During the remainder of the first stage of labor, Heather's contractions began to slow down. She dilated to 9 centimeters, and an anterior lip of the cervix remained as an obstacle to complete dilation. She struggled with the lip, then dilated completely. As she began pushing, Heather actually pushed the baby back rather than forwards, and her anterior lip reappeared.* She responded to encouragement by claiming exhaustion and the inability to go any further. An hour of pushing showed no progress in labor, and Heather became increasingly dependent and adamant about her inability to push her baby out. She predictably began talking herself into distress over her exhaustion at her effort, imploring others to tell her what to do. Her contractions dwindled and remained ineffective as she beseeched others to help her.

---

*This unusual occurence (pushing the baby back into the uterus, rather than forwards) has taken place with 3 other women in my experience all of whom also experienced significant ambivalence towards the unborn child, and all of whom (including Heather) were single-mothers.

Because the attending physician and I knew Heather's conflicts and fears, but mostly because we were familiar with her personal growth process, we were able to recognize her physical process as related to her psychological process. We understood that the more we encouraged her, the more dependent she became, and the more ineffective her contractions were. We knew that it was important to withdraw our presence from the room in order for Heather to focus on her own resources, rather than looking for outside help. We hoped that this would stimulate a sense of responsibility for action, for resolution, as this was her personal growth process as it had become known to us in the process of psychotherapy. We told Heather that we would be leaving the room for a half hour in order to give her time to herself to rest and to have a chance for effective contractions to begin before moving to regular labor and delivery for an intravenous hormone which would stimulate contractions. Heather was left with a supportive hospital nurse whom she did not know previously. Her friends left with us. Heather did not ask for instructions from the nurse, as she did not know her as well. After resting for 15 minutes, she asked the nurse to put on a record she had brought with her. She then got on the floor, with only the support of the bed for her upper body, her knees on the floor. She had previously been unwilling to try this position when we had suggested it earlier. She pushed for 10 minutes. When we came back into the room, Heather had pushed her baby part way down her vagina. She was making good progress. The baby's heart tones were good and were listened to by the nurse periodically.

When we came in Heather again stopped labor, began asking for instructions, insisting she did not know how to do it. We sensed that she was de-focusing from her own resources and the work at hand. We again left, to sit in a nearby room, telling Heather we would be back in a half hour. The nurse came to get us in 10 more minutes as the baby's head was showing and crowning of the head was imminent. We quietly came into the room. Heather continued to push her 7 lb. baby girl out, with no tears on the perineum, and turned around to greet her newborn. She bonded to her baby in the next several hours after birth, and left for home the next morning. Heather continues to feel her bond to her baby grow much stronger as her initial ambivalence towards mothering yields to her acceptance of this new responsibility. Her identity continues to form and re-form in the postpartum period, creating a place for herself as mother within her feminist perspective. She was able to re-define womanhood to include both strength and motherhood.

An aspect of Heather's experience which bears further elaboration is the increased choice available within a holistic framework. By this I am referring to the greater opportunity for resolution towards a normal labor and delivery that was available to Heather through a psychophysiological approach to childbirth.

In addition to knowledge of her psychological growth process, we were familiar with Heather's "performance anxiety" around the birth experience, and the fact that this anxiety increased when she was with people she knew, as compared to people she did not know. In our absence, her anxiety lessened, as the hospital nurse was someone unfamiliar to her. She did not need to struggle with preoccupation to please others with whom she had a relationship. Beyond a point, support from us and from friends began to intimidate rather than facilitate focus on the work of labor. Perception and timing in terms of this type of psychological intervention were delicately balanced in order to prevent Heather from sinking into the role of "victim".

The ability to include the psychological as well as the medical in labor assitance improved the possiblity of normal outcome for birth. It provides a wider spectrum of choice which includes change and growth as an ever present, ever creative potentiality.

Heather had classical uterine inertia, which traditionally leaves but one medical choice of intervention—hormonal intravenous solution. However, with a psychological approach involving the connection of the mind-body processes, another avenue of choice was open; one in which Heather could have the kind of birth experience she desired, and so feel the control she had of her own life. Such experiences leave women with strength and confidence as well as create an optimal environment for maternal-infant bonding.[5] Bonding in this case was crucial for Heather, since an unfulfilling birth experience in which she would feel out of control of her body, could have had a negative effect on her beginning relationship with her child. Intense ambivalence and negativity about her identity as a woman and mother could have reappeared. For Heather, particularly, labor and birth was a time of creative stress and crisis transformed to fulfillment. The gains in maternal attachment and confidence that are witnessed at a birth experience in which the mother has been an active participant and afterwards feels very positive, cannot be underestimated. For some women the birth experience is more crucial to the bonding phenomenon than for others, depending on the individual's personal background, beliefs, and attitudes. For Heather, birth was a delicately balanced point in time of terrific impact. A positive birth experience in which she felt in control was significant in bonding her to a baby she had felt ambivalence towards in pregnancy. The greater the mother's ambivalence, the greater the importance of a positive birth experience to enhance the bonding phenomenon and to increase feelings of maternal-infant attachment.

Had Heather not been able to push her baby out, and had she received medical intervention she would have received emotional support and help for continuation of the process. At that point, her body would have been clearly too exhausted to continue the process without physical medical intervention. Emotional support at this point in time would have also been crucial, as there is absolutely no guilt or blame to be attached to needed medical intervention. Non-separation of mother and child would be even more important under such conditions, as the mother would need every opportunity to bond with her baby to increase the likelihood of experiencing her birth as a positive fulfilling event; one in which she was rewarded with her baby's presence after the difficult labor. Had this happened for Heather she may still have developed her confidence in mothering skills, but it would have taken longer, and would have been more protracted a process during post-partum. Postpartum depression would also have most probably been prominent. It is important to nurture and accept a woman at her own place of development, as is always true in the psychotherapeutic process. Should physical medical intervention be necessary, such acceptance and support is even more important. Delicately balanced within the framework of this nurturing and acceptance, is the knowledge and ability of the birth attendant to create opportunity for the woman herself to achieve her own goals. Too often in medical practice, midwives, physicians, and other health care workers think of their duty as one of saving. Emotional support and caring should be ever present, however, without taking the power away from the client herself. The more skilled the health professional is in creating opportunity for change, whether it be a labor in which uterine intertia develops, or an illness, the greater the possibility for personal growth and fulfillment. The use of psychophysiological integration techniques and the skills of a good psychotherapist in a health care setting opens the possibility for clients to experience the ability to choose their own reality, and to interpret their experience with their body in a meaningful way. Bodily experience does affect the psychological growth of a person. Psychological beliefs, attitudes and conflicts are expressed in bodily conditions and processes.[6] Such is the basis for holistic health.

Many individuals interested in improving the medical model espouse a belief in holistic health care in which a state of mind is given equal importance to the physical state. Many health care workers proclaim the importance of a giving, caring relationship but fail to obtain the training in psychology that would enable them to remain free of the "savior" position in which they have been trained. The caring relationship is half of what is needed. The other half is the training to recognize psychological process and personal responsibility. When people are given and can accept personal responsibility for their bodies, they accept their own power. It is with this sense of power that they gain control of their own bodies and lives.

Without this psychological awareness and the skills to lead clients at their own pace towards this source of power in themselves, many well-meaning health workers easily fall into the position of "savior" or rescuer. [7] The "savior" is also the robber of the client's personal power.

In the context and meaning of holistic health care as I define it, it becomes important to meet a client at whatever level of personal responsibility she/he is at, and to use what skills I have learned and developed to work towards giving the client his/her own power back. As healers, we seek to guide others towards healing themselves. Dependency on the health professional is often the beginning of the relationship, as it is often in psychotherapy. But through the relationship, the dependency is transferred back to the client, with the sense of personal power being born within the client. The relationship can then continue to flower into a system of support and nurturance which the client uses as needed as a resource for life challenges. In this way, clients educate themselves from the resources that are available in the form of both medical information and stimulation for increasing their own self-esteem and confidence for problem solving.

An emotional, caring relationship, in which respect for the client creates an environment in which self-esteem can grow, is an important ingredient in the relationship between health professional and client. An extremely skilled health professional, one who can move one step ahead of the client in the process of development of the client's inner resources, is an essential ingredient to the relationship as well. These ingredients—the skill to provide emotional support and acceptance of the client and guidance towards personal power—provided the opportunity for Heather to effect a change in herself which allowed her to give birth in the manner she desired.

Other diminutive, or augmentative qualities are too numerous to mention here, but include stability of the home environment, and relationship of the couple. The family system, with its rules, dictated roles and patterns of interaction[8] can play significant roles in augmenting or diminishing an individual's inner resources for labor, birth and parenting.

In addition to the approach to life and attitudinal resources presented, environment also should be evaluated. The present living situations, especially as regards the couple's relationship, can either augment or diminish a woman's existing psychological resources to handle stress. Supportive, nurturing relationships and relatively harmonious living conditions can strengthen an individual, while disharmony and constant struggle can lead to severe distress if not resolved. Here again, evaluation of such stress is always individual. Couple disharmony or single motherhood is distressful to the extent that it is experienced as such by the individual woman.

Couples' and family counselling to increase communication can greatly relieve stress and facilitate smoother functioning of the family system. Such counselling can be suggested to couples in childbirth classes as a way of preparation for labor, birth, and integrating a new baby into their lives. The childbirth professional should give permission and support for such intervention when the need is apparent.

A woman's inner resources can be developed throughout pregnancy, as it is a natural time of growth and reflection. The move towards natural birth is a part of the greater woman's liberation movement. To gain control of our lives, of our destiny; to validate ourselves through the authenticity of our experience; such is the desire of the woman choosing to birth naturally. As women, we want to experience our bodies throughout the process, to claim the power of birth that is ours, to respect it, and to grow within ourselves as we integrate the natural forces. Hormonal secretion and neurochemical responses which accompany the emotional turbulence of birth and postpartum reflect the actual life transition of a baby into physical form. Hormonal and neurological changes serve to facilitate emotional responses such as maternal-infant bonding. Bonding becomes the healing phenomenon for the transitional stress of redefining the family to include the addition of a new member. Thus, a hormonal reaction of the body effects a psychological response in the maternal-infant relationship, which in turn affects the ease of acceptance into the family.

Psychophysiological Integration

This brings us to an important principle contained within the framework of childbirth preparation as psychotherapy, and illustrated in the above case example: the integration of mind and body. Our bodies are a source of information in the form of physical biofeedback. Unhappy, dissatisfied mind states are reflected in body posture and movement. Our feelings can be read in our movements, as we physically relate to the world in context of our perception of ourselves in relation to others.[9] The importance of getting familiar with our bodies and of making such information accessible to ourselves is reflected in the body experience of birthing. The more a woman can cooperate with her body to push her baby out, the smoother the journey through the vagina becomes. Being aware of tension, being able to relax and to let go of tension in a particular part of the body, becomes the process of yielding and working actively with the physical labor of birth.

Relaxation training becomes an important part of childbirth preparation, but it must be linked with an active frame of mind to be effective. Relaxation as such develops into strength. Active relaxation can be taught throughout prenatal classes, as well as the philosophy of active participation in labor. As women become aware of their bodies, they can begin to recognize anxiety and fear as it is translated into body tension. In this manner, women can be educated to the mind-body link and the relationship of life style and mental state to physical health. In holistic prenatal care, individual, couple, and family counselling is encouraged when it is deemed necessary to facilitate deeper understanding of the psychological state, and when it can catalyze change in the family system and the individual woman's self-perception towards the manifestation of strength and capability necessary for birth. There is ample opportunity for the childbirth educator and health practitioner to give permission to those women needing extra counselling to seek it out.*

---

*This becomes easier within a holistic team approach in which a woman does not have to seek outside services to obtain counselling. This is the advantage of including a mental health worker as part of the health team.

Fear, and especially unrecognized life stress, can constrict the life breathing passageways, as well as the birth-giving passageways of the body. Visualizing the labor process with positive suggestion for ability to birth can be instrumental in inspiring a change of attitude in particular women. Both guided visualization and playing audio recordings of labors which include pain as a part of the process act towards systematic desensitization[10] of phobias and fears of childbirth. Both women and men can be led through the birth process as vividly as possible, giving rise to confidence by working through fears and labor rehearsal while engaged in deep relaxation and guided imagery. A birth visualization takes place in the first class of the series of late holistic childbirth classes which begin at the 7th month of pregnancy. Getting to know the baby through body awareness in pregnancy becomes a very powerful reinforcer for the labor process. Positive imagery may also be employed to change behavior and symptoms such as morning sickness. Cassette recordings of the visualization of labor may be used for individual women to re-learn a healthier concept of childbirth when needed. The birth visualization will be explored in a later chapter devoted specifically to the evolution of this psychophysiological integration technique. I have experienced much success with turning breech babies (in the last few weeks before birth) to vertex position through the use of this technique. This phenomenon has been achieved through relaxation, visualization, and psychotherapy combined into what we (of the Holistic Psychotherapy and Medical Group*) have termed a psychophysiological integration technique. We have found mind-body integration to be a most powerful means of effecting change on the physical level.**

Recognizing those at risk for developing complications in labor due to an inability to cope with stress and/or pain can be advantageous for being able to work to prevent complications in labor. Holistic childbirth classes as I have designed them

---

*Holistic Psychotherapy and Medical Group is a private group practice in Berkeley, California.
**The lower uterine segment is controlled by the autonomic nervous system. In individual cases, mounting inner tension due to conflict about birth, mothering, or other influences can result in an involuntary tightening of the lower uterine segment, which is controlled by the autonomic nervous system. Involuntary tightening of the lower uterine segment (similar to the involuntary tightening of blood vessels, which some people exhibit under stress, resulting in heightened blood pressure) can make it impossible for the fetus to engage its' head in the lower pelvis or to settle in a head-down position, resulting in a breech presentation in late pregnancy.

I have had an 80% success rate with women 35 - 40 weeks gestation, utilizing psychophysiological integration to facilitate the relaxation of this lower segment and the change to vertex presentation of the fetus. This success contrasts dramatically with the medically expected spontaneous turning rate of 20%. More will be written about this phenomenon in another book.

emphasize a woman's ability to recognize stress in herself and to identify it, in part, through conscious body awareness. Slow deep breathing, sound, and relaxation are presented in classes in the framework of increasing body awareness, which is necessarily present in birth. Slow, regular breathing insures the body of the life-giving oxygen needed, both for baby and mother. It also releases the body to respond to hormones without interference of panic or distrust. As a woman learns about her body and trusts in it, she can let herself be guided by the body knowledge available without resisting it. Relaxation is taught as a way to get to know the body and to be comfortable and accepting of the body experience of pregnancy, labor and birth. Release of sound as an integral experience of breathing serves to cement the relationship of mind to body. Creating sound through breath stimulates the intense inner focus needed in childbirth. Breathing, sound and relaxation as such become centering devices which work primarily *through the relationship of a significant other.* It is then the emotional support person (labor coach or husband) who serves to nurture strength, confidence and self-reliance in the woman throughout the labor process. Use of sound in psychophysiological integration will be described in Chapter V.

Labor and birth become a time of learning; of learning more about one's self, one's partner, one's view of life. As we live, so do we give birth. Growth and development are reflected here, microcosmically, as they are in life. To become more of who we are in pregnancy, offers more depth of perception in birth and can continue onto another plane in parenthood if we let it. Labor as a time of learning is a major emphasis of the classes. As we approach a given situation with an orientation of learning more about ourselves, we are more open to the psychological adjustment necessary for the situation at hand. In this framework, a woman can be encouraged in her own creativity for finding a meaningful way of working through labor.

The classes help to prepare a couple for the intensity of labor and provide them with centering techniques which work through relationship and in the framework of mind-body integration. Slides and particularly audio cassette tapes of labor and birth present labor as a realistic challenge to grow through.

After classes are finished in late pregnancy, a psychological openness must settle into each woman's life, as she deals intimately and uniquely with her relationship with nature. How she will relate to the incredible energy of the life force she is creating within her as she gives birth to physical form, is still unknown. The ability to develop her inner resources and prepare the physical arrangements must reach a level of closure. New psychological receptivity immediately before the labor must be accompanied by a sense of calmness and expectation for the unknown. Acceptance of the approaching meeting of body and mind and a sense of being simultaneously prepared yet unprepared constitute a necessary transition after classes. Women who have not yet reached this developmental phase of late pregnancy may be encouraged to do so with private, individual attention. Confrontation of fears in a very concrete manner may catalyze the necessary development needed at this time. The peacefulness associated with this final state of openness is reflected from a state of inner psychological development which has rendered the woman confident in herself. This self-acceptance and strength allows for meeting an unknown situation (particularly true of first babies) such as labor openly and creatively and without the anxiety usually accompanying journeying into the unknown. While it is true that physical and psychological mapping of the journey may reduce some anxiety, it is emphasized in the classes, realistically, that no amount of preparation but the experience itself can prepare them for the actual intensity of birth. This concept of acceptance of the unknown is an important aspect of good preparation.

Adequate preparation should leave a couple calm and strong at the gateway to the unknown. They have seen and examined their inner reflection in this pregnancy—their fears, desires, and expectations. They have strengthened their inner resources for dealing with stress and the unknown in life. Labor is an unknown. A woman does not know what her labor will be like. Classes do not prepare her for what her labor will be for her. So she is entering the unknown and knows it. She is prepared only to meet the unknown in herself and is confident in her ability to look to herself for resources needed during her labor. This has been her preparation—that only she can give birth and that she must look to herself for strength, stamina, and active participation in birthing her baby. If she has learned this, she has learned much more.

REFERENCES

Chapter 2

1. Simonton, O. C., Simonton, M. S., and Creighton, J. *Getting Well Again.* Los Angeles, J. P. Tarcher, 1978.

2. Butler, N. R. and Borham, D. G. *Perinatal Morality: The First Report of the 1958 British Perinatal Morality Survey.* Edinburgh, E. & S. Livingstone, 1963.

3. Gadpaille, W. *Cycles of Sex.* New York, Charles Scribner and Sons, 1975.

4. Freud, S. *Three Contributions to the Theory of Sex.* New York, Dutton, 1962.

5. Peterson, G. and Mehl, L. Some Determinants of Maternal Attachment. *American Journal of Psychiatry*, 135:10, Oct. 1978.

6. Simonton, O. C. and Simonton, S. *Stress, Psychological Factors and Cancer.* Los Angeles, J. P. Tarcher, 1977.

7. For further information on the psychodynamics created in a rescue situation see: Steiner, C. The Rescue Triangle. *Issues in Radical Therapy*, Vol. 1, no. 4, Fall 1973.

8. For further information on rules within the context of the family system see: Satir, V. *Peoplemaking*, Palo Alto, Science and Behavior Books, 1975.

9. Lowen, A. *Bioenergetics*, New York, Penguin Books, 1976.

10. Desensitization is a technique which couples relaxation with the visualization of progressively more anxiety provoking scenes in order to decrease anxiety. Further information may be found in: Bandura, A. *Principles of Behavior Modification.* San Francisco, Holt, Reinhart, and Winston, 1969.

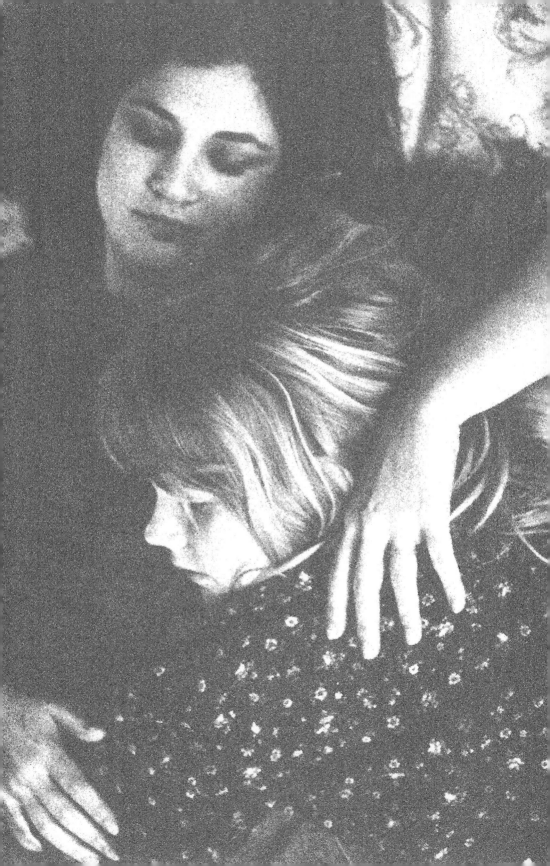

Chapter Three

Early Pregnancy Classes

THE FIRST THREE months of pregnancy are barely noticeable to others, but to the pregnant woman, this can be one of the most stressful trimesters, especially for a first pregnancy. Enormous body changes are taking place. A woman's hormonal system is adjusting to maintain the pregnancy. Increased progesterone and estrogen serve to nurture the developing fetus in the corpus luteum, while simultaneously the placenta is rapidly being formed to nurture the developing fetus through the nine month gestation. The placenta is fully formed and functioning by the 10th week of pregnancy. Body temperature rises as the metabolic rate is increased, and a 40% increase in blood volume occurs which calls for an increased amount of work for the cardiovascular system. In the first trimester the basic foundation is formed, as well as the adjustment of the woman's body state, to carry the fetus to the normal 9 month gestation. Such adjustment will continue throughout the pregnancy, but is most striking in the early months when the initial shifts in body hormones, metabolism, and cardiovascular activity occur.

It is during this time of enormous work that others often have no clue that the woman is undergoing such biological metamorphosis. Fatigue sets in very heavily for many women, especially if they expect themselves to "not feel any different". Morning sickness is also common in this phase of pregnancy.

In my model of Holistic Prenatal Care early pregnancy classes are designed to validate this work being done. Such work is "invisible". It is done unconsciously without need for deliberate direction. It is nonetheless physical work. Education about how the foods she eats provide the pregnant woman with the resources she needs for the physical work of making a baby become paramount. Diet counseling can be achieved in a group setting in the form of a class. Responsibility for keeping a diary of the food eaten throughout the week, adding up calories and determining the distribution of vitamins, protein, iron, calcium, and other nutrients should be part of the client's participation in early prenatal classes. In this manner, women begin very early to become aware of the importance of their own actions and how these actions affect physical health. It should be emphasized that only the woman can eat the food needed. No one else can do it for her, just as no one can give birth for her (and do it naturally).

Lifestyle, by way of diet and nutrition, points the way to a woman's control of her body. She decides whether or not to live in a manner which promotes health. Smoking, diet, sleep and exercise habits are all primarily under the control of the person doing them. Feelings of not having control over such habits can be recognized early and support for exploration of the underlying psychodynamics or stress which may be exacerbating such symptoms can be given. For example, economic reasons for poor diet may in fact have roots in deeper conflict. A low income family in which a husband's alcohol is of higher priority than the quality of food eaten in the household, is suffering a family conflict deeper than the economic consequences of alcoholism. Another example is of a woman who sees herself as worthy only as long as she continues working outside the home, even though she is suffering extreme fatigue and lack of appropriate diet and exercise which contribute to a mood of depression during her pregnancy. Such a woman may be suffering fears of identity change in motherhood which hold her back from enjoying a healthy pregnancy. In order to validate work done on a biological level during early pregnancy classes, parents-to-be are shown color slides of the developing fetus from conception through the first trimester, and then on to later pregnancy and full term gestation. Information on the inner work of making a baby is made available, as well as a connection to the mothering process already underway.

As a woman nurtures and carries the unborn fetus inside of her, she is already mothering on a biological level. She is nurturing the baby, giving it what it needs through her own body system. The blood, oxygen, and nutrients are carried through her placenta, through a single blood vessel in the umbilical cord, and into the baby. Wastes are carried away through two remaining blood vessels in the umbilical cord out to the placenta through the mother's body to the outside world. The mother is physically mothering on an automatic, unconscious level. Through birth, a woman travels from mothering on a purely biological cellular level to mothering on a conscious, deliberate level of raising a newborn to adulthood. The point of birth becomes a meeting ground of intuitive body knowledge and conscious, logical mind process.

Women are taught during these early classes that the blueprints for giving birth exist within the body. They are also brought in touch with their own body knowledge. As she continues the process of creation of the baby inside of her, the individual woman's body holds the knowledge to its creation. A woman is making a boy or girl inside of her, or twins as the case may be. Her body is not confused. She does not make a boy, if in fact it is to be a girl, or a girl if it is to be a boy. The blueprints are laid out in the body. In early pregnancy classes women are encouraged to feel their body experience, and to trust their body knowledge. There is a part of them that knows if they are making a girl or boy just as the time of conception is immediately noted biologically, and so too are the blueprints of gestational due date within the realm of a woman's body knowledge.

Women are encouraged to become more familiar with their bodies both through physical exercise and through relaxation exercises taught early in pregnancy. It is not the type of relaxation and physical exercise so much as the underlying body awareness through the experience of the physical focus of the exercise that is important. Normal exercises in pregnancy are referred to in the early classes, such as those that can be found in Elizabeth Noble's *Exercises for the Childbearing Years.*[1] In addition to specific physical exercises, it is emphasized that women should be maintaining a level of daily physical activity which is slightly challenging to them. Physical stimulation will strengthen the cardiovascular system and ready it for the work of labor. Physical strength and stamina are emphasized, and building body strength increases body awareness. Again, the woman is taught that only she can ensure that she will benefit from physical exercise, as a result of her own determination to incorporate it into her schedule. Individual responsibility and choice with regard to physical exercise is emphasized as another example of control over physical health and the greater possibility of a healthy normal delivery.

The more comfortable a woman is with her body the more familiar she is with it, and the less inhibited she is capable of being in childbirth. Lack of inhibition in labor and birth enables her to follow her body rhythm, by participating fully in the body experience. Vocalization of body sensation, particularly pain, is encouraged as it is congruent with the outward body energy of birth. Women are encouraged to squat, to become psychologically comfortable with open legged positions. Perineal massage is taught in these two early classes to ensure adequate stretching of the perineum during birth in order to reduce the possibility of tearing. However, more importantly, the perineal massage serves to acquaint or further familiarize women with their genitals, their vaginas and to experience awareness of these parts of the body in pregnancy and birth. Perineal massage can be done by the father-to-be as well, as such gives permission for sexual exploration to be a part of the pregnancy. Changes in hormones can cause changes in labial size, elasticity of the vaginal tissue, as well as changes in color and texture of the vagina. Women are able to experience these changes in their bodies during pregnancy and to validate such body transformation as healthy and creative.

Perineal Massage at Home

The man (or woman herself) is instructed to gently massage in a circular motion around the vaginal opening, including the labial and clitoral area. Such massage is physically aimed at promoting an abundant blood supply to the perineal tissue to lessen the occurrence of tearing during childbirth. The man (or woman, if she is doing it herself) should then rim just inside of the vagina, moving one or two fingers around the inside of the opening, gently stretching the vaginal opening particularly nearest the perineum (the area between the anus and vagina). A massage oil should be used to minimize friction and increase stretching of the tissue. Oils such as wheat germ, cod liver, or vitamin E are recommended as all of these oils contain vitamins A, D, and/or E which are healthy for skin tissue. Perineal massage several times a week is recommended in early classes, and increased to daily during late classes.

Perineal massage can open psychological doors, too. A woman is able to become familiar with her vagina and more comfortable with the awareness of her own sexuality as it relates to birth. Her body is accessible to her, as it needs to be in birth.

Sexual Validation in Pregnancy

The majority of women seeking natural births in the United States today are already well aware of the emotional and spiritual aspects of such an experience. However, few give the physical experience of birth the attention it deserves. Without the body experience, birth becomes an unnatural or anesthetized experience. For this reason, integration of the physical into the psycho-emotional aspects of pregnancy and birth should be emphasized in these early pregnancy classes. Being able to feel ourselves as sexual, as connected to our bodies and to feel ourselves as physical strength in the form of muscle and bone, creates in us a sense of trust in our bodies. One goal is to develop within the pregnant woman a sense of trust in her body and to deepen the trust she already has. She will then be able to believe in her body process as labor unfolds rather than be frightened or alienated from it.

Sexuality needs to be emphasized as a part of our natural given biological right. The freedom to enjoy sexual pleasure during pregnancy, and in our lives in general, is addressed in early pregnancy classes. The classes serve as opportunities for a group of pregnant women and interested partners to explore issues of sexuality. Birth is an expression of our sexual nature and to give birth is to express oneself sexually. Pregnant women need support in identifying themselves as sexual. Sexuality is not an act, but a part of life. To include the genitals in the acceptance of the body becomes a sexual expression of identity. Pregnant women are stimulated towards positive identification with their womanhood. Support for strength in womanhood, as well as yielding, is conveyed through an attitude that includes preparation for childbirth within the definition of women's sexuality.

Relaxation

Relaxation exercises are begun early in pregnancy. Again, this seems to familiarize a woman to her body, and her control of each part of it. It also brings her in touch with the changes in her body over the course of her pregnancy, keeping her in touch with the development of the fetus. In addition, relaxation serves to decrease anxiety and to increase the ability to learn and to confront fears in pregnancy, birth and parenting. Relaxation is used towards the beginning of a class to facilitate inner reflection of anxiety or fears related to pregnancy, labor and birth. As class members relax, psychological defenses are let down and people are more vulnerable to their emotions. Group discussion of expectations, fears, and feelings about childbirth are encouraged. Special attention is paid to confronting fears in childbirth which can take the form of denial. Denial of pain is often a cloak behind which fears of inadequacy lie. It is important to deal with denial of pain within the context of the group and on an individual basis if it continues through to late pregnancy classes. Confrontation of fear is mild in early classes, as many women have spontaneously confronted themselves by the time they reach later pregnancy. Fear confrontation will be dealt with further in the framework of the later classes.

At least one set of relaxation exercises should be aimed specifically at developing awareness of the couple relationship. Focusing on the sensation of touch to the exclusion of other senses can be an introductory experience to the concept of touch as nonverbal communication. Simply instructing each partner to massage the other partner in a way that will convey a particular emotion can open doors of communication around the issue of relating during labor and in general.

Instructions for one specific exercise is given as an example:

Touch

"Sit cross-legged on the floor with your eyes closed, facing your partner. Without words simply take turns exploring your partner's hands. Specify who will go first. Now explore your own hands (3-5 minutes) with eyes closed.

"Now touch your partner's hands playfully with eyes still closed (5 minutes). Play with each other's hands. Now touch each other's hands seriously. Be serious with each other's hands (5 minutes). Now touch each other's hands tenderly. Be tender with one another's hands (5 minutes). Share feelings and insights of this exploration with one another and with the group."

An awareness of how they related to one another, what they like about how they relate, and what they would like to change about how they relate in touch, can have far-reaching effects on the couple's awareness of the manner in which they are presently relating to one another.

Sensitivity to touch is taught early as a means of communication to the laboring woman. Learning what she means when she says "firm" or "soft" can be discovered now. In addition to touch and massage as a means of labor support, it is important for the woman to learn to touch her husband or labor support person. In this way she can learn how to better communicate her own preferences.

As couples take one another for granted at times, pregnancy is a good opportunity to remind them of tenderness with one another.

Being tender with your partner helps to maintain open doorways of communication which are important in labor and in life. When communication is open, a woman is free to be less inhibited during birth. Both partners are better able to express openly their expectations, fears, and desires of labor and birth, of one another during labor, and of one another in parenthood.

Additional exercises can be assigned for homework. Massage, sensate focus[2] or any other form of exploring one another's bodies without sex as the goal can be recommended. Additional homework exercises are to facilitate the awareness of touch within the relationship and of how each touches the other and wants to be touched by the other, and to encourage open communication and expression of feelings. The sexual act itself should be prohibited during the time specifically set aside for the homework exercises, so that touching does not become goal oriented. Such homework should be given after the first early class. Insight, expression of feelings, and further discussion can continue at the second early pregnancy class which should be scheduled one week from the first. This allows time for reflection and understanding of the couple relationship as it is defined in the present. Redefining the couple relationship, as needed or desired, can be facilitated at this time. Again, the awareness of choice and responsibility is emphasized with regards to communication and couple relatedness.

Early classes serve to introduce inner contemplation about labor and birth as being a time of expressive and active work. The concept of relaxation is couched within a framework of active emotional participation in the labor and birth. Preparation for birth as including pain as a part of the labor process is introduced here.

Diet, exercise, relaxation and sexuality are major points of focus at this time, all aiming towards building and nurturing trust in the body. Education to body knowledge and process in pregnancy becomes the cornerstone for confidence in childbirth and mothering in the near future. The blueprints are there. The body knows how to create the fetus and how to give birth; the mind can learn from it. With the aid of body hormones, a woman proceeds after birth to mother in a conscious, deliberate manner. After birth, the mother may still feed the baby with milk nutrients from the body, but she is doing so deliberately by putting the child to the breast, rather than unconsciously through her placenta as in pregnancy. This meeting of body and mind during birth creates and releases enormous energy for growth, as it is an opening through which a new soul emerges and new relationships are begun. These family relationships continue to expand personal possibilities for infinite variations of psychological growth, change, and development.

The view of pregnancy and birth as a journey inward has begun at the end of the first trimester. Birth becomes an opportunity for psychological growth and an event to which a laboring woman relates intimately and uniquely, weaving a learning experience all her own. Like pregnancy, birth is a time of great fluidity when psycho-emotional conflicts are also very salient. As such, it is an opportunity for seeing one's self in clearer light than ever before. To use this opportunity can be as rewarding as the gift of the newborn child. Women are educated to this rewarding opportunity in the early pregnancy classes. They are guided inwards, setting the groundwork for late classes which aim at developing inner resources specifically for the task of labor.

REFERENCES

1. Noble, E. *Exercises For The Childbearing Year.* Boston, Houghton & Mifflin, 1982.

2. Kaplan, H.S. *The New Sex Therapy.* New York, New York Times Books, 1974.

Section II
Holistic Childbirth Preparation

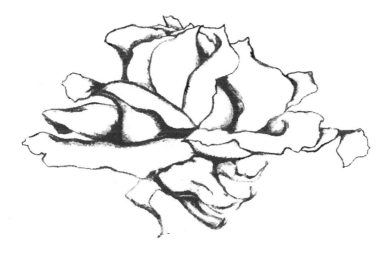

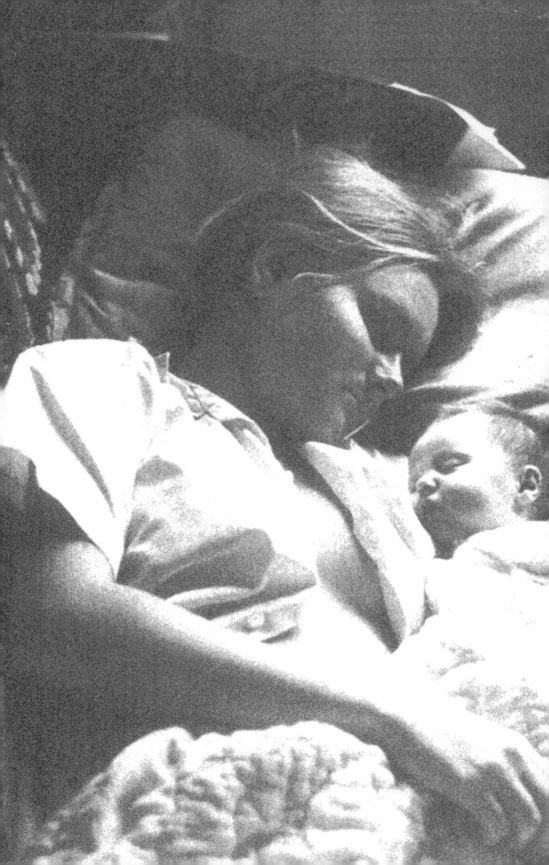

Chapter Four

The Inner Map of Birth

DURING THE FIRST class of the late pregnancy series, couples are taught an inner map of birth in the framework of a relaxation induction and birth visualization.

Both men and women are guided through a progressive relaxation process, beginning with attention to breathing. They are directed inwards, gradually gaining awareness of the body and their ability to consciously direct changes in muscular tension. After the relaxation induction is completed, couples are guided through the birth process from an internal journey from the womb, outwards through the cervix, and coming down through the vagina. In this visualization of the birth process, women and men gain an experiential knowledge of birth from an emotional level, before they learn the physical anatomy, or what I refer to as the outer map of the birth journey. Yet, at the same time, the physical journey of birth is explained as a byproduct of the experiential visualization.

It is important for the pregnant woman to understand the concept of power and force in relation to uterine contractions. In labor, contractions push the baby's head down, hard on the cervix, letting the cervix stretch from the force of the contraction, and the woman needs to yield to such power. A woman needs to be able to own that power as it comes through her, to add to the strength of the contraction, especially in second stage during pushing, while simultaneously relaxing and yielding to the force she is helping to create in order to birth her baby. This combination of strength and yielding can be best taught through the encouragement of vocal expression of the body's sensation. The woman can express pain by active, long, powerful vocalizations, which can wed her to the force of the contraction without need for denial or resistance to it.

Once a woman accepts her right to be uninhibited vocally, she may or may not actually use sound in labor. The ability to be open to any manner of release which she may want to express during labor is the desired result. However, simply stating that a woman should allow herself the right to such uninhibitedness is not enough. Acceptance of this ability to become uninhibited in labor occurs as a woman hears and practices "letting go", in this case through the use of vocalization in childbirth classes.

The following is an example of a relaxation induction and birth visualization as done in the first class of the late series. Attention should be given to the fact that, once relaxed, people are more susceptible to suggestion. Much information can be absorbed on this experiential level which also reaches a form of hypnosis in which hypnotic suggestions of opening to birth, contracting down after birth for the placenta, and contracting the uterus after the placenta is born in order to prevent hemorrhage are given. Interpretations of what are direct and indirect hypnotic suggestion[1] are given as well as other pertinent interpretation as necessary throughout the narration.

Instructions are given for couples to lie comfortably on the floor with eyes closed. Throughout the relaxation induction, vocal dynamics play a key role. It is important for the childbirth teacher to speak in a regular, conversational tone near the beginning, letting the voice become quieter and speaking slower with a sing-song quality as the relaxation process progresses. The words should be spoken slowly, but with pauses and phrasing for emphasis. Emphasis is instrumental in formulation of hypnotic suggestion. Hypnotic suggestion is suggestion given in a state of deep relaxation, phrased in such a way as to decrease the probability of resistance to the suggestion, and to increase the probability of its acceptance.

Part I
Relaxation Induction

"Listen to your breathing. Let your breathing become a little deeper . . . Now become aware of what is happening biologically as you breathe. You are taking air into your body, taking oxygen to each and every cell in your body, and as you breathe out, you are breathing out what you *don't* need. You are breathing out carbon dioxide, toxins in the air, as you effectively filter out all that you don't need. Take in what you need, and for the women, as you breathe in oxygen, you take oxygen into your placenta, through the cord to your baby, as you breathe out, you breathe out what you don't need, what your baby doesn't need . . . and now I'd like you to take this a little further. I'd like you to imagine being able to take from the air, from your environment, what you need for yourself and breathing out what you don't need; stress, worries, tension. You can give yourself the right, just *now*, to breathe out any' tension you've been holding onto during the day, during the week. You can just *begin* to allow yourself to breathe out tension from your body."

Interpretation:

The intimate association of mind and body has been made through the immediacy of breath. Breathing out what you *don't* need on a biological level, is already an indirect hypnotic suggestion to breathe out "other" things the person doesn't need. These are not verbalized until later, i.e., tension, worries, stress. In this manner class members can be led indirectly to release tension, bypassing resistance more successfully.

By validating truths that everyone takes for granted about the body (breathing in oxygen, breathing out carbon dioxide) clients can be led into a relaxed state involving letting go of mental attitudes (worry, stress) through the body.

Emphasizing words that are underlined creates an unnoticed command (to relax, NOW) which is then responded to automatically. Emphasizing *beginning* avoids resistance due to performance anxiety.

The intimate body connection with the baby has already begun, and with each breath, an awareness of the baby has already been formed as an unconscious association. Because of the undeniable truth that the baby receives oxygen with each breath, whatever else is said during the following phrase or two, is also accepted with little resistance.

The relaxation induction continues, now progressively moving through the body, and development of imagery begins, so as to create a more intense focus, or hypnotic trance.[2]

* * *

"With your next breath, imagine breathing out any tension from the left shoulder, all the way *down* through the arm to the elbow . . . through the lower arm *down* through the wrist and hand and right out the finger tips. So that the arm can just begin to let go. It doesn't have to do anything. It can just begin to relax more and more with each breath out.

With the next breath, breathe out any tension from your right shoulder all the way *down* through your arm to your elbow . . . then breathe out from the lower arm all the way down to the wrist and hand and right out the finger tips. So that this right arm too can just begin to relax, to let go. It doesn't have to do anything."

Interpretation:

The word "down", repeated, sometimes emphasized, creates a rhythmic quality which relaxes and soothes, and also alludes to going deeper into a hypnotic trance, which is merely a deeply relaxed state of mind and body. "Down" also refers to going down through the birth canal, which is where "down" leads to later in the birth visualization.

* * *

"And now take your attention down to your left hip, once again, breathing out any tension from that hip all the way *down* through the thigh to the knee. And you can imagine what the thigh looks like on the inside . . . the blood vessels, the muscle, the nerve network, the bone. With each breath, oxygen is carried to those blood vessels. And you can consciously begin to direct your breath to that part of your body, breathing out any tension from that thigh muscle and letting sensation build at the knee . . . and build, and build, until finally it washes through to the lower leg, breathing out tension from your calf muscle all the way down through the ankle and foot and right out the toes. So that this left leg doesn't have to do anything, doesn't have to go anywhere. It can just be allowed to become more and more relaxed, going deeper and deeper with each breath."

Interpretation:

Imagery has now been introduced. It is the beginning of a deeper trance state, or relaxation. "Consciously directing" breath into a part of the body gives the indirect suggestion of ability to gain control over the muscular relaxation at will. Thus, relaxation technique is being learned as something that *can* be consciously achieved through breath. Negative suggestions of "not having to do anything" or "not having to go anywhere" has the effect of relieving performance anxiety and acts as permission for relaxing.

* * *

"With your next breath, breathe out any tension from your right leg, all the way down through your thigh to your knee, letting the sensation of the breath build at the knee... and build... and build, until it spills over into the lower leg, washing away any tension that stands in the way of that relaxation. Breathe on out through the ankle and foot and right out the toes. Again, letting this leg become more and more relaxed with each breath. It doesn't have to hold you up. It can just be given the right to let go . . . to just be."

Interpretation:

The vague word "sensation" usually avoids resistance, due to its ambiguity. Sensation can be very individual, and so internally, the individual is able to match the command easily. This is more effective than to give a more direct word such as "pleasant", or "still" which might alert the class member to an opposite feeling he or she is having in the knee. The fact that a "sensation" is felt is proof of suggestibility, and again resistance is bypassed, and some sensation which is unique to each person is in fact produced in the knee. Learning and response of an experiential nature has already begun in the relaxation induction, prior to beginning the birth visualization itself.

* * *

"And now let your attention focus in the throat, and as you breathe in, you can just let the throat become more and more loose, more and more open. So that your breath can massage the inside of your body. With each breath, feel the breath create more and more room as your throat becomes relaxed and open. The throat is very important in childbirth as it is very connected to the vagina. So just let the air open your throat more and more with each breath... And now follow your breath down into your chest, feeling your chest rise and expand as the air comes in . . . and fall as you breathe out. Follow your breath all the way down through the chest, on down through to the stomach, making more space inside you as you breathe . . . more room for each internal organ in your body —

the heart, lungs, stomach . . . to find their natural healthy position in the body (directed to the women: "and adjust as necessary in pregnancy . . . labor . . . birth").

"And now as you breathe out, breathe out any tension, or knots of tension from the stomach, so that as you breathe out your stomach can become very calm, very relaxed, much like a calm peaceful lake. Your breath can loosen any knots from the stomach, letting it become more and more relaxed with each breath.

"And now for the women, just let your breathing continue deeper, and as you breathe in through your throat, let yourself imagine breathing out right down through the vagina, letting the walls of the vagina relax more and more with each breath out. Breathe right out through the vagina letting it become very relaxed and open, loose, very very open for birth. So that you are breathing in through the throat and all the way down and out through the vagina creating a very clear, open passageway for birth.

Interpretation:

By moving down inside the body and increasing the amount of imagery, attention has now come to the womb, though not yet directly. Opening for birth has been anticipated by starting with the throat relaxation. The deep breathing for birth is being taught through the relaxation induction. Breathing in through the throat and out through the cervix and vagina during labor is encouraged directly in later classes. However, it has already been experienced and explained in this first class. I gave an indirect hypnotic suggestion to adjust or yield to pregnancy, labor and birth in the form of internal organ adjustment to labor and birth. "A clear passageway for birth" is linked with the relaxation itself and breathing.

The relaxation induction continues to include the urethra and anus, developing into a deeper state as each person travels down the spine, sliding down each vertebrae with an internal breath massage. By this time, even the most resistant will usually be lying relaxed and in a receptive state for learning. Then, after attention to the urethra and anus, and following the breath down the spine has occurred (in a similar manner to the above narration) the induction moves on towards the birth visualization.

* * *

"Now focus on the back of the neck letting the sensation of relaxation spread up your scalp, letting any tension fall away from your head, on the lines of your hair, right out onto the floor. You don't need it (the tension). Let the sensation continue down your face, letting your eyebrows become farther and farther apart, drifting farther apart, all the way down over the cheeks, nose, mouth, jaw, right down to the throat again. Once again, letting the throat become more and more relaxed and loose."

Interpretation:

A cycle has been completed. The throat was marked as an important place earlier, and we now return to this area, ready to go on to a deeper level.

Part II
Birth Visualization

"And now for the men, I'd like you to give yourself the right to imagine a clear glass window in the uterus through which you will be able to follow your partner's breath as she breathes oxygen into the baby you are both creating.

"Now for the women, follow your breath down through your throat, chest, all the way down through to the uterus, to your womb. As you breathe in, you carry nutrients right through the placenta, through the cord which has 3 blood vessels. One blood vessel carries nutrients to the baby, while 2 carry waste products away from the baby through the cord and out through your system, through your breath. Give yourself the right to imagine what it looks like inside the womb. The color of the uterine walls, the texture of the placenta, the waters . . . and the baby floating, cradled in the pelvic bones . . . and hearing the heartbeat through the waters, and right now, your baby is very developed, perfectly formed, just waiting to be finished. The baby is covered with soft hair which will fall off most of its body before it is born. Fingernails and toenails are growing, the baby now has a unique hand print and foot print all its own. It looks very much like a baby, your baby. And there's a body knowledge in each woman that knows a whole lot about this baby whether it's a boy or a girl, because the body is creating one or the other (adjust as necessary for twins, etc.), when labor and birth will occur, because conception was known biologically. Just as the body knows full well how to make this baby, you also know how to birth. And right now you are one, connected, physically one with your baby. I'd like you to take a moment to just become that part of the body right now, which is your baby. Give yourself the right to 'pretend', just as you did as a child, fantasizing what it would be like on the inside. (PAUSE) Whatever learning needs to take place can spontaneously occur, as you do this, but *without* any effort on your part. You can be curious . . . and explore. And you can learn from the body, without any conscious awareness; any changes that need to occur can spontaneously develop . . . as needed . . . for labor . . . for birth . . . for parenting. Just enjoy the body knowledge, the ease of learning . . . relaxation."

Interpretation:

Many truisms are given about body knowledge which create conscious agreement in the person undergoing the induction. This agreement is then carefully linked with suggestion for learning about birth, for changing, developing in any way necessary for labor, birth, parenting. Emphasis on tone of voice relays an importance to certain words, which are automatically picked up on an unconscious level; such as *inside, without effort* (to reduce resistance), *curious, explore, learn.* Interspersed throughout these suggestions are instructions to *just relax,* that a person need not be aware consciously what is going on. With this kind of instruction, a kind of hypnotic trance can develop, whereby a person is most susceptible to learning through visualization, because conscious beliefs or attitudes which might limit learning or limit the imagination, are occupied with double bind instruction, i. e., do learn, do imagine, but without effort, just enjoy, spontaneously. [3]

The visualization then proceeds to labor and birth. An understanding of labor can be realized, and suggestion for normal labor and delivery can be given.

* * *

"Now, from the baby's point of view, just imagine what the cervix looks like, where it is. And take yourself forward in time, as if through a time tunnel, to the time of labor and birth. When your baby will be ready for the journey, completely ready to come out and into your arms. You can feel contractions coming throughout the day, but now they're beginning to get harder and stronger and you can feel the baby's head, and see it, pressing very very firmly down on the cervix. So very firmly that the cervix is beginning to stretch, to open . . . and you feel another contraction starting, like a car coming from way down the road in the distance and it's coming closer and closer and the contraction is getting harder and harder and your baby's head is pressing harder and harder down on the cervix, and you can *feel* the baby's head coming down, and you open, and you open and then the contraction begins to fade, and fade . . . and you rest, and your baby rests. And you sink into an even deeper relaxation, where your resources are endless, and you gather strength for the next contraction."

Interpretation and Continuation of the Visualization:

There is significant quiet for approximately 45 seconds, and then a continuation beginning with the next contraction, with similar visual imagery and suggestion. *Most important is the use of voice dynamics in this imagery.* The voice must build in pitch, in intensity of volume, in speed, creating a very real sense of urgency and focus in the experience. Women oftentimes comment afterwards on feeling the urge to push or sensation of pressure with the visualization experience.

Rhythmic rests and building intensity through imagery and vocal dynamics to simulate a contraction proceed so that this has been done approximately 4 times, with the suggestion of contractions coming again and coming and going, to create the illusion of time passing in labor until, with the 4th time, the baby's head is coming right through the cervix, diving down, down, coming right through, as the cervix is fully dilated.

A rest is again given and then the visualization proceeds with an increased intensity to push as the contraction builds.

* * *

"And now you can feel it coming again.* This time very hard and fast, building and building, and your baby is diving right down, down, towards the opening of the vagina. And you can feel the strength and power of the uterus, pushing and pushing, contracting down, harder and harder, and you let it happen. You open to the incredible strength, and you push and push and you can feel the baby's head, right there in the vagina, coming down and down and then the contraction begins to fade, and you let it

---

*I often make use of the imagery of the ocean, the building of waves to simulate contractions and the imagery of the bottom of the ocean in between contractions to embed hypnotic suggestion for the development of resources for handling labor.

fade and the baby comes back just a tiny bit, ready for the next surge forward. And you rest and your baby rests. And your baby is getting very massaged, very stimulated for breathing."

Interpretation:

Again, vocal dynamics build and reach a peak, until the word fade is spoken. Then the vocal dynamics slow, to suggest rest and silence. Within the content of the imagery for 2nd stage are suggestions for labor to be perceived as very healthy, normal, despite its great intensity. Mothers sometimes fear the strength and intensity of contractions for the baby's sake. Here, it is asserted that labor is intense and powerful *and* very healthy for the baby. An association of health with the intense sensation of labor contractions is a conditioning that encourages an absence of fear and tenseness for the labor process. As fear reactions tend to stop labor, this is a very significant yet subtle connection to be made in the context of the visualization.

* * *

Suggestion for strength is given and emphasized during 2nd stage as this is when women often times become very tired, especially if they have led themselves to believe in a "transition" phase. The use of the word "transition" is avoided as it creates the myth that labor is "downhill" from that point on. In fact I emphasize a need for increased strength and activity during 2nd stage and teach a woman that her labor is not over until the baby is born. She can expect a continual increase in the intensity of the experience to the time of actual birth itself, whereby the physical intensity is then transferred to an emotional level, and the "birth high" which has been documented ensues.[4]

A total of 3 contractions is usually the content of 2nd stage in the visualization although again time is not defined as a number of contractions, since contractions "coming and going" is also inserted in the narration of the birth visualization.

During the final contraction there is an emphasis on panting and letting the perineum stretch so that the baby can be born without tearing. Another contraction happens for the shoulders, and the mother "hears" her baby breathe, then "feels" it against her skin, in her arms, "sees" it looking up at her.* As the baby is

---

*"Hearing," "seeing," and "feeling," are spoken as embedded hypnotic commands which involve the participation of the secondary visual, kinesthetic, and auditory cortices of the brain, connecting through the limbic system. Visualization is effective through the actual creation of memory linked to the experiential process. A more thorough explanation of this subject matter will be offered in a forthcoming book.

born another contraction is described as the woman imagines her uterus clamping down very firmly to give birth to the whole placenta. Suggestion is given for the uterus to continue contracting down very hard and firm (to prevent hemorrhage). The couple is then encouraged to just enjoy the fantasy of holding and touching their baby and this involvement is deepened by the added fact that "this is not very far away, just another 6 weeks or so. It's a very, very real image and will be happening in only a little more than a month or so."

Couples are encouraged to indulge in the fantasy, which is drawing nearer and nearer to present reality, of becoming parents to this new baby.

After a few minutes it is suggested that the image fade into the future and they are re-oriented to the present, to the baby inside, "not yet ready for the journey, but knowing full well the journey when the time comes." Imagery of the baby at its present stage of development in the uterus is then narrated, then focus is shifted to the breath, to the body relaxation, to the sensation of being the center of the room they are occupying at the time. Suggestions are given for feeling refreshed and facilitating any learning as needed, as time passes.

Through the visualization process, the anatomical information of the labor and birth process has been given on an experiential level. This is what I term the "inner mapping" of birth, as opposed to "outer mapping" which occurs in the next class, using the birth atlas and textbook pictures for explanation of the process. Visual imagery learning of the birth process has the advantage of being more meaningful to the individual, as it is the particular person's individual imagery which has been facilitated. Therefore, the physical process of the cervix thinning and opening and the baby moving through the vagina which stretches as the baby moves down the vagina, as well as the explanation of the physical process for the baby (stimulating it for breathing, etc.) has all been taught as a part of the emotional experience of the visualization. Exploration of feelings and the experience of focus in birth is made available through the experiential nature of the process. Men are given a more intimate understanding of labor than is usually the case in childbirth classes.

In addition to education of the physical process, and more significant, are the indirect hypnotic suggestions to have a normal, healthy labor and delivery. In some ways, a woman giving birth for the first time has some of the advantages through the visualization experience, that a woman who has given birth before has from direct experience. A more realistic expectation for the intensity of the labor increases the woman's resources to deal with labor at the time.

An emotional learning of a normal labor and delivery has occurred, and this emotional learning itself is a hypnotic suggestion for healthy labor and birth. Fear is minimized, which in and of itself, can minimize abnormal labor patterns, and maximize any voluntary control over the process which would increase the chances for a normal delivery (i.e., active and effective pushing in 2nd stage and relaxation for more effective dilation).

Indirect suggestion given for learning and development, as well as changes needed for labor and birth, can activate resources in the person (i.e., a woman who perceives herself to have a low pain threshhold can learn to tolerate pain). Any psychological blocks for birth (i.e., ambivalence towards the baby, perception of self as too weak for birth) may be encouraged towards resolution as the person is in a receptive state. The suggestions for learning and change are non-specific enough to become personal for each individual's interpretation and act to mobilize the development of resources necessary for any particular woman for birthing.

Still, such development is always in the hands of the woman herself. All we as childbirth professionals can do is to facilitate any inner development necessary and attempt to encourage the movement of conflict toward resolution.

Breathing and Sound for Focusing Energy in Labor

After a relaxation induction, women can more readily learn slow breathing for labor as the air-giving passageways are relaxed enough for them to feel the sensation of breath coming through the throat and into their bodies.

The intent of the slow, deep breathing is to create a sense of focus which is achieved through the connection of visual imagery and kinesthetic sensation in the body. This type of focus in a very relaxed state is also the essence of a hypnotic trance. This trance state is characteristic of the level of awareness in which we make contact with ourselves and experience meaning in life. It is an everyday occurrence, and happens spontaneously whenever our attention is absorbed in one focus, i.e., reading a book, writing a letter, daydreaming, creating art pieces (music, dance, painting). The object is to reveal to each person her/his own ability to voluntarily enter this creative state, and to use it for direction of energy, in this case for birthing. A woman can learn to effectively direct her energy in labor through breath and sound as mechanisms for focusing attention. Once learned for birth, this ability to enter the creative trance state at will is of tremendous value. It is in this state we can visualize what we want for ourselves, and it is in this state, through direction of energy outwards, that we form it.

Deep breathing in the context of childbirth classes is learning to feel and direct energy in the body.

Instructions for Deep Breathing Focus in Labor

Have partners sit cross-legged on the floor facing one another. Partners are instructed to simply breathe deeply for the duration of one minute (in through the nose, out through the mouth, making an aperture with the lips), counting each breath, simply to become aware of how many slow breaths they take in a minute. Four to eight breaths per minute is the range wherein most people fall, and it is considered a normal, healthy range. Women breathing less than 4 breaths a minute may be holding onto the breath, creating unnecessary tension, while women breathing over 8 breaths per minute probably are not breathing deeply enough. Counting breaths per minute is then repeated, but this time with the labor support person following and breathing as the woman breathes. The husband or support person then counts and follows each breath the pregnant woman takes, with his/her own breath.

At this point instructions are given to once again do the deep breathing together, this time creating aspirant sound as they breathe outwards which can be easily made by adjusting the tongue in the mouth in such a way that air coming out makes a whispery or whooshing sound. The word "shh," when we are asking someone to be quiet, utilizes this type of sound. However, deep breathing for childbirth preparation is done with a slight aperture of the lips on the exhale, creating a small opening through which the air is directed, thus the sound is more of a wind-like sound, "sssssssssss".

Instructions continue:

"Breathe in through your throat, yielding to the air as it enters your body, creating more room inside. As you breathe out (with the aspirant sound) feel yourself sink down, feel the relaxation of the body as it expels the air, gently collapsing downwards, feeling it all the way through the vagina and out, just as the breath comes out."

The aspirant sound which accompanies the breath has the effect of increasing the depth of breath right down through to the diaphragm muscle as the breathing occurs. The diaphragm muscle is very important in childbirth. This muscle sits high on top of the uterus of a pregnant woman in the last months of pregnancy. As it is used for breath and sound, it assists in pushing down on the uterus, helping to provide muscle strength needed for pushing a baby out, especially in 2nd stage of labor, but also in pressure which acts as a natural aid to first stage dilation. The quality of the sound is very important and can be taught in the classes as a controlled, directed energy which aids the body in birth, as opposed to a shallow screaming, which does not originate in the diaphragm, but in the vocal chords and chest area. Therefore, deep breathing down to the diaphragm is essential, as sound originating from the diaphragm does result from an open, relaxed throat. Hysterical screaming is a dispersal of energy and results from a closed or tight throat, chest or stomach.

Teaching deep breathing with utilization of the diaphragm for sound also affects the body's overall relaxation. The sound itself creates a focus of attention for childbirth, and also insures the open air passageways conducive to relaxation and letting go. It is almost impossible to make sound from the diaphragm (singing, calling a lost dog) and tense the vaginal muscles. Use of sound does insure a clear passageway for birth, if the quality of sound is the kind originating in the diaphragm. More will be said about the use of sound in birth in Chapter V. For now, it is important to understand that use of the diaphragm in deep breathing does in fact open the throat, chest, pelvic muscles, vagina, urethra, and anus. Sound that increases the use of the diaphragm is taught in the classes.

"Now just close your eyes and continue slow, deep breathing, imagining what it looks like on the inside of your throat as the air comes in, creating space, as the throat opens, all the way down through the chest, like a very open tunnelway." Breathing out (with aspirant sound) follows the natural relaxation of the collapse of the upper chest as it yields to the pressure in the diaphragm which deflates the last bit of air and sound in the body.

The need to take in air with the next breath cycle is automatic, and increasingly the diaphragm begins to be used to suck air into the body as well as expel it. Expelling the air with use of the diaphragm is on a small scale exactly what will be happening as women push their babies out. During labor, the intensity and magnitude of this exercise is increased many fold. If this breathing exercise were able to be increased to an intensity similar in labor, urine and feces would be eliminated, which in fact is what happens during labor. A baby would also be directed out, and on a much smaller scale, this exercise is of the same energy direction as that of birth. The same physical processes are occurring internally—use of the diaphragm and opening the throat, chest, vagina, urethra, and anus through the breathing exercise. The focus of attention, or creative trance state is also apparent. Having women practice this breathing exercise puts them in a similar mind state as that needed for effective labor. The following scale illustrates the continuum of this creative trance state of mind and body.

The Creative Trance State

low intensity		high intensity
	Mentally	Physically Initiated
Spontaneous	Initiated	Activites Necessitating
Daily	Physical	Complete Absorption
Activity	Activity	into the Physical Process

$$\overset{\displaystyle 0 \qquad\quad 25 \qquad\qquad\quad 50 \qquad\qquad 75 \qquad\qquad 100}{\vdash\!\!-\!\!-\!\!-\!\!-\!\!-\!\!\mid\!\!-\!\!-\!\!-\!\!-\!\!-\!\!-\!\!-\!\!+\!\!-\!\!-\!\!-\!\!-\!\!-\!\!-\!\!+\!\!-\!\!-\!\!-\!\!-\!\!-\!\!-\!\!\dashv}$$

Daily activities of varying intensity; i.e., daydreaming, reading, writing, playing, listening	Directed activities: deep breathing, artistic creation (music, dance, singing, painting)	Sexual orgasm	Labor and Birth

The process of pregnancy from conception to birth is a process of ever continuing outward expression of energy, from internal creation to manifestation in physical reality. As deep breathing of the nature described is practiced, women develop their ability to focus and direct their energy in birth. Women are asked to practice throughout the week and to bring questions to the next class. However, it is emphasized that there will not be a lot of "practice" taking place in the classes as the classes are a place of instruction and learning. The practice must take place on an individual's level of responsibility. This is emphasized in the beginning to encourage the self-motivation which is necessary for any learning process. Too much practice during class time leads to a state of dependency on class time for assimilation of learning which presumes an amount of time not available in classes. If a woman is given the respect and the responsibility for carrying out practice on an individual basis, the class material has a greater chance of becoming meaningful to her in her everyday living experience. Women are informed that the ability to focus attention and direct energy for birth comes out of a daily practice which cannot be simulated in classes. Only they can do the work , just as in labor and birth.

I have had great success with this approach and the vast majority of women do in fact take the practice seriously, availing themselves of the opportunity for self-directed growth of a psychological nature as they gain ability to enter the creative trance state at will.

In this first class men and women alike share their respective experiences of the visualizations and of their experience of the pregnancy thus far. Group interaction is encouraged and a feeling of travelling together for the course of the next month of pregnancy is facilitated. Many of the couples have also seen and interacted with other parents-to-be during the course of the prenatal classes and may continue to see one another after birth. There is ample opportunity for development of support groups and friendships given encouragement by the childbirth teacher to do so. However, even if couples have not seen one another prenatally or do not become resources for one another after birth, there remains an atmosphere of warmth and closeness during the classes as emotional experience is shared and accepted.

REFERENCES

1. Grinder, J., Bandler, R. and DeLozier, J. *Patterns of the Hypnotic Techniques of Milton H., Erickson, M.D.* Vols. I and II, Cupertino, Meta Publications, 1977.

2. For further explanation of hypnotic trance see: Rossi, E. and Erickson, M. H. *Hypnotic Realities.* New York, Irvington, 1974.

3. For further explanation of therapeutic application of the double bind consult: Bateson, G., Jackson, D., Haley, J. and Weakland, J. Toward a Theory of Schizophrenia. *Behavioral Science,* 1:251-264, 1956.

4. Lang, R. *The Birth Book.* Felton, New Genesis Press, 1977.

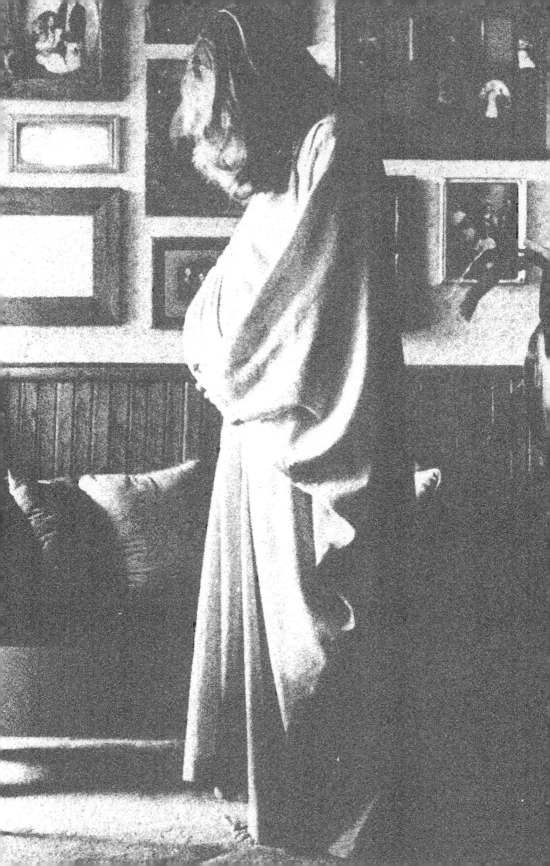

Chapter Five

The Outer Map of Birth

THROUGH THE BIRTH visualization, women and men have learned the birth process. They have learned it emotionally through personal symbols constructed by their own creativity. The visualization process has also illustrated the mechanics of labor. The following attitudes for healthy delivery have been taught through the experiential process:
—Labor as a powerful and healthy force
—The baby as resilient and ready for the transition to outside the womb
—Labor as a healthy process for the baby, stimulating the baby for breathing.
The significance of the above messages cannot be underestimated, as all of these concepts influence a woman's attitude towards labor. A belief that babies are delicate influences the mother's expectations for labor and her images of how she will respond to contractions. Some popular books currently on the market present the baby as an incredibly delicate being who is bound for inevitable trauma by being born. The attitude of sensitivity to the baby is laudable; however, the indirect message to the parents that the baby is fragile presents to the laboring mother a conflict between the power of contractions and the "gentleness" with which she is supposed to be birthing, according to these books. If the woman has been indoctrinated to the necessity of birthing quietly and gently, she can come to an unbridgeable gap between her romantic image of a gentle birth and her own physical labor, alienating herself from her body and the labor process. The underlying belief she is fighting is that birth is innately a traumatic process. She is then put in a position of fighting the labor to make it a gentle, non-traumatic process. The

complementary belief is that the baby is too fragile to be born, too fragile for the intensity of contractions. The solution for the woman can be to lessen the contractions to a more "manageable" level, rendering contractions ineffectual but gentle: uterine inertia.*

A case history illustrates this point:

Laurel was a 27 year old woman expecting her 3rd baby and planning a home delivery. She indicated desire for a "LeBoyer"[1] birth, which she interpreted to be quiet and gentle. Her first child had been born with anesthesia 8 years earlier, and her second baby, born 6 years later, was a natural birth in a hospital setting. Laurel expressed negative feelings about both deliveries. She associated her negative feelings about the second birth with the hospital environment. Her desire for home delivery grew out of her beliefs that labor would be easier at home and less traumatic. Throughout her pregnancy and prenatal classes, Laurel clung to the belief that labor would be easier at home, easier for both herself and her baby.

Laurel went into labor on her due date. When the birth attendant arrived at her house her cervix was at 2 centimeters dilation.** Laurel was encouraged to go about her daily activities at a relaxed pace, and the birth attendant went home to await a call from her that she was in hard labor. Laurel did not go about her usual activities, but remained awake most of the night, sure that her baby would be born at daybreak. In 24 hours, Laurel was 3-4 centimeters, and beginning to feel that contractions were becoming "too strong". She was encouraged to focus her attention on hard labor, on letting the contractions build to sufficient strength for birthing her baby.

Laurel lit candles and put on a flowing white nightgown, settling herself on a quilted bed to the sound of soft Indian music in the background. She felt she was now ready for her gentle home birth. Laurel remained making very slow progress to 6½ centimeters. During this time, the birth attendant had noted the increased strength of contractions at the times she would use the

---

*Uterine inertia is a complication of labor in which the uterus stops contracting, or contracts only mildly.

**Dilation refers to the measurement in centimeters of the opening of the cervix. The cervix needs to dilate to 10 centimeters in order for a full term baby to pass through it.

toilet. As the time grew near to go to the hospital for Pitocin,* the birth attendant suggested she sit for a while on the toilet, in the chance that contractions could start up again in this position. Laurel did this, with her contractions starting up again and becoming strong, until she would return to her candle-lit bedroom where contractions would again become ineffectual and weak.

Finally, the birth attendant asked her to remain on the toilet, at which point Laurel complained that this was not her "idea" of a home birth. Laurel was confronted with her unrealistic expectations for labor at home to be easier, less painful, and romantic. She complained, but remained on the toilet as this was the only place her body could labor effectively. In the bathroom environment, Laurel temporarily removed herself from the romantic beliefs about home birth which had alienated her from the labor process. She began to vocalize, yelling on the toilet, bringing herself through to second stage. At this point the music in the background ended, and no one put it back on, as the focus of the environment had changed to make way for birth. With some lights turned on, Laurel was able to return to the bedroom, actively pushing her baby out. Unconcerned about "quiet," "gentle" birth, Laurel pushed very actively, yelling through the pain of the contractions, birthing a 7 pound healthy baby girl.

Laurel realized afterwards that much of the negativity she had associated with her second child's birth had been the sensation of pain which she had attributed to the hospital setting rather than labor itself.

Her beliefs that the baby was delicate, and that she wanted to birth the baby gently and quietly did not include pain. Her understanding of "LeBoyer" style birth did not give her the ability to adjust to the power of labor.[1] The only resolution for integrating her beliefs into the process was to alter the process to fit her beliefs. However, once her beliefs were revealed as limiting ones for her birth, she was able to learn at a crucial point in her labor an attitude which was necessary for freeing herself to follow the natural force of her own labor.

Early in prenatal classes, the attitude towards birth as a positive and aggressive natural force which is both intensely powerful and stimulating for the baby is taught. Women are then free to adjust to the intensity and pain of labor without holding back for fear

---

*Pitocin is a synthetic hormone (to replace the natural hormone, oxytocin) used for augmenting the strength of contractions during labor, and is used in cases of uterine inertia.

the labor process will hurt the baby or cause trauma. Within the context of belief that the baby is resilient, that labor is meant to be powerful, and that the power of contractions includes pain, a woman can adjust to her own experience.

By the second class women have been educated about birth through an inner visual map of their own making. The mechanics of the process and attitudes conducive to normal delivery have been communicated through guided visual imagery. Although the visualization is guided, the actual personal imagery of any individual is unique and intimately symbolic. This is both the potential and the limitation of the group imagery process. The potential for learning through images is great. As labor is described, an assurance that the cervix can open gives an individual permission to imagine the cervix opening in her/his own mind. However, the kind of cervix that is imagined will be unique to the individual's beliefs and self-image. In a group visualization, learning is the primary goal, and spontaneous change in limiting beliefs can occur through the birth visualization. However, the extent of such learning cannot be measured, except in individual one-to-one visualization, in which the therapist can get verbal feedback on an individual basis as to the specific quality of imagery. Because of this limitation of the group setting, women who may exhibit conflict or present limiting beliefs for birth are encouraged to come in on an individual basis for help with mind-body integration. Mind-body integration in this context is defined as changing beliefs which could interfere with the woman's adjustment to labor. Beliefs are emotionally learned concepts which can be unlearned or re-learned most readily in the same emotional state in which they were originally learned. Behavioral psychologists define this concept as state dependent learning.[2]

When I work with women individually, I often use the technique of visualization (along with indirect hypnosis) to facilitate an emotional re-learning process. During this process, which may take place through a series of therapy sessions, I work with the woman to identify beliefs through her imagery, facilitating work through the emotional state in which a particular limiting belief was learned to a point at which the opportunity for a more constructive belief for giving birth may be learned in the present in the same emotional state. The following example illustrates the potential for this learning process as it relates to birth, motherhood, and life in general.

Farrow lived with her husband of 1½ years and her son, age 9, from an earlier marriage. During part of her pregnancy her husband's daughter, also age 9, resided with them. There was some distress on Farrow's part in defining the family, particularly with a new baby due in 7 months. Family therapy focusing on the above was under way when Farrow realized her need to resolve her feelings about her first childbirth experience. Because of guilt feelings about her labor, birth and early mothering experience with David, her son, she found herself unable to discipline him. She behaved towards David as though she were guilty of a crime which could never be forgiven; was consistently trying to "make it up to him" by pleasing him in any way he desired. Consequently, David suffered from a lack of parental limitation which increased his manipulation of his mother. He also manifested this lack in behavior problems at school.

Farrow's guilt, which limited her ability to discipline David was not the sole source of David's behavior. David was also expressing much of the disorder and mis-communication present in the family system at that time. However, one necessary step towards effective communication and a clear definition of family rules was Farrow's ability to set limitations for David. As Farrow became aware of her belief in "making things up to David" she came up against a limitation in herself which required resolution of her inner conflict about the first childbirth and postpartum experience. Rather than attempting to gain this resolution through atonement to David, Farrow began to look to herself for the answer.

Through a relaxation/visualization process, Farrow was guided back in time to the days immediately preceding her labor and birth of David. As she re-lived this experience in the present, Farrow described herself as passively trying to deliver at home, by not going to the hospital when her bag of waters began leaking, and labor started. She expressed a desire to remove herself from the hospital setting, but she had no planning or preparation for home delivery. She was hoping it would just "happen," easily and with little effort. She had not told anyone of her desire for home delivery, except her husband who was totally unsupporting of the birth in general. Farrow began having mild contractions which, after four days of ruptured membranes (broken waters), did not increase in strength. Finally, she was admitted to the hospital and labor induced.

Farrow described the labor process as so painful that she had to remove herself from her body. Each time a contraction began,

Farrow found herself looking down on her body writhing in pain.

Through weekly sessions, Farrow came to a realization that her process of removing herself from a situation when it became too stressful was a pattern she had learned as a child growing up in her family with an alcoholic father. She had learned to remove herself from her house when her father became drunk and violent. While this had been a very healthy pattern of adaptation in her childhood situation, this same pattern had persisted in adulthood, limiting her ability to adjust to situations in which flight was not her best option.

During a second visualization in which Farrow experimented with changing her childbirth experience, she found herself believing that God would give her only the amount of pain she could handle. As Farrow reflected on this belief which had surfaced during the visualization experience of her last labor, she became aware that she had limited the amount of pain, as she clung to her belief that God would not give her too much pain. When her labor was induced, the pain was seen as coming from the outside, as being forced on her, and she adapted by removing herself from her body, as the labor-inducing drugs flowed through her veins.

Farrow was guided through a visualization of herself giving birth, this time letting herself feel the pain of each contraction. The result was a vision of herself as a whole woman, accepting the pain and work of labor. She was able to visualize herself as responsible for the process, and as relying on her own resources rather than relying on a God who would give her a labor without pain. She re-learned emotionally the concept of responsibility, which allowed her to remain in her body during labor. She was able to cry as her baby was born, granting herself the joy of keeping him close to her rather than the separation which had ensued in the hospital. She was able to grieve the loss of that moment in the past, and to grant herself a right to it in the future.

During a third visualization, Farrow became aware of how she had remained passive in her relationship with her ex-husband, removing herself from the responsibility of motherhood. As she visualized her postpartum course with David, she became aware of how she had limited her responsibility, becoming entrapped in a prison of being "taken care of" by her former husband. She had permitted her husband to banish her from the house for a week in order to "break her" of picking up her 2 month old son every time he cried in the night. Through her passive removal, Farrow had gotten herself into a very painful situation, in which her own motherhood was denied by an extremely jealous husband. As she struggled with her husband over her rights as a mother, Farrow decided to divorce him and become the mother to her child that she wanted to be. It took her one year to acquire the courage to leave her husband. Her guilt for not having been the mother she had wanted to be to her newborn continued for the next 8 years.

Through weekly therapy sessions, Farrow continued to gain awareness of her beliefs about fathers, her own father, and David's father. She was able to view her belief system more objectively, and had begun to identify new beliefs which she wanted to take the place of the old ones that had limited her.

Through a fourth visualization, Farrow was able to say goodbye to her ex-husband, to feel sorry for him, but not feel responsible for his pain. Without this responsibility, she did not need to remove herself from the situation of dealing with him about visitation and bringing up David. She was able to see herself grow strong and sure in her motherhood, taking responsibility for her own pain, but not the pain of her ex-husband. Taking responsibility for her child, she gained the right to motherhood.

Farrow was able to transfer this new belief in herself as a strong mother to her relationship with David. She could trust her feelings of what was right for him, and take responsibility for setting limits.

Farrow's behavior changed. Significant was her ability to limit David's visits to his father to a consistent pattern, rather than succumb to sporadic and unpredictable urgings to see his father, against Farrow's better judgment. As she was able to believe in her strength and responsibility, Farrow did not remove herself from stressful situations with David, but offered instead a consistency and predictability to their relationship, working through disagreements with consistent discipline as necessary.

The result was a much calmer, happier David. Within two months his behavior at school had noticeably improved and his relationship with Farrow was more rewarding. He began showing interest in the coming baby, responding positively for the first time to the prospect of a new brother or sister. David appeared more relaxed as he felt the security of his place in the family.

As Farrow was able to resolve her own difficulties concerning her guilt over David's birth and early mothering, she was able to become the mother David needed her to be. Through counselling sessions using visualization for learning and re-learning, Farrow was able to identify beliefs and attitudes which had affected both her childbirth and her ongoing mothering experience with David.

Through the emotional turbulence of these sessions emerged a woman free to be a mother. Farrow no longer waited for her ex-husband to grant her motherhood. She no longer waited for God to handle her struggles and pain. She no longer removed herself from David when he needed her most, at this time of re-definition of the family (both through Farrow's second marriage and through the pregnancy). She accepted her responsibilities as she accepted her strength. She was no longer the victim of her past, but a woman choosing to change the pattern of passive victimization which she had helped to construct. As she did change her past, through the visualization process, seeing herself give birth, accepting the pain and labor, and seeing herself say goodbye to her ex-husband before he could rob her of her rights as a mother, Farrow's attitudes towards herself changed. She was no longer ridden with guilt, passive, and dominated by her nine year old son. She became instead the woman who had given birth in the manner she wanted to, and had stayed with her child at the age of two months when he needed her by him .

For Farrow, the beliefs and patterns of adaptation uncovered in the birth expressed the same style of living which now affected her mothering. True to the premise of this book, Farrow had given birth as she lived her life at that time. By re-living this event, Farrow was able to identify patterns of coping which limited her in birth, in mothering, in life. She was able to apply the change in belief that would have increased her chances of normal delivery with David, to her present relationship with him. As she lives these new changes in herself, she is preparing for her next birth. The learning that has taken place in preparation for birth and in an attempt to define the family for the birth of the coming baby, has had long-reaching effects on Farrow and the family. She was able to use her pregnancy, both as an opportunity for growth and as a time to resolve hidden conflict. The pregnancy became a magnifying glass into her past, and as she was able to change in the present, to come to terms with her past, she affected her future. Her new-found strength and responsibility will affect everything she comes in contact with, including her relationship with David and the birth of her second child. The same kind of emotional learning takes place in classes, but not usually on as deep a level, for if an individual does not recognize resistances, there may be a need for individual intervention which group visualization does not encompass. The use of visualization within the context of psychotherapy is a tool for creating change which can be faster than the traditional Western analytic approach. Emotional learning rather that intellectual insight, is emphasized in the visualization process.

Getting feedback from the group on the visualization process and facilitating discussion of the personal imagery can further learning about the mechanics of birth, and possibly identify those women who might benefit from individual therapy sessions to further explore birth-related beliefs or resolve crucial issues.

Birth Atlas

The birth atlas[3] is a pictorial account of the birthing process, depicting the descent of a full term baby through the vaginal canal and out into the world. Pictures of the cervix pulling back to make way for the baby as the baby's head is applied to the cervix facilitate discussion and understanding of the normal birthing process.

The birth atlas can be used to cement the learning process through representation of an outer map of birth, presenting pictures of the baby's descent, but only after inner images have already been developed. Labor and birth as a process, rather than a set of stages, has already been experienced through the visualization. Progress through the birth atlas is usually fairly rapid, as most questions have already been answered in the visualization. The visualization has presented a framework in which to assimilate further learning, which can then take place more rapidly and with greater meaning for the individual. The birth atlas in the second class acts as a solidifying agent for the learning that has taken place the week before. Once the inner map of birth has been explored, the outer map, as described in the birth atlas is readily comprehended.

With the mechanics of birth consciously realized, the class is ready for further experiential preparation for birth.

Audio Cassette Tapes of Labor

The power of sound should not be underestimated. The power of an effective contraction in labor should also not be underestimated if a woman is to be prepared for birth. During the second late class in the prenatal series, after the birth atlas has been shown, the women and their partners experience two contractions by ear.

A tape of a woman in hard labor is played. The tape used is one in which intensity of a contraction can be heard as it builds, peaks, and wanes through the vocalization of the particular woman. This process of listening through intense contractions and the silence in between gives the class members a sense of the immediacy, the intimacy, and the intense focus of hard labor. Class members are then encouraged to react, release, contemplate, and in general to respond in their own way to the auditory experience. The sound of the first two contractions can open people to their fears, their expectations, and may also loosen limiting beliefs about labor. Members are able to share their feelings, learning more about themselves through their reactions and the reactions of others to the tape. The intensity of the sound rarely fails to bring couples into increased intimate contact with one another, and especially for the women, into intimate contact with nature. Fears can be explored with the childbirth educator, who acts as both teacher and facilitator of an emotional resolution of fears in birth.

Members are also guided by the teacher towards an assimilation or an accomodation of pain in labor into a healthy, meaningful experience.* The concept of pain as healthy in labor has been begun to be taught on an experiential level, as the members discover their emotional reactions to the sound of a woman in labor.

Through this auditory experience, members are unable to deny pain as part of the labor, as it can be identified by ear. The attitude of acceptance and normalcy that is exhibited by the teacher (especially if, in fact, it was her labor, or one she was present at) is a *powerfully hypnotic role model.* When the class members have heard the two contractions, and if they are having difficulty accepting the pain as healthy, they are temporarily disoriented, groping for the stability again of their own perceptions and beliefs. The greater their distance from belief of pain in labor as healthy, the greater their disorientation. The disorientation itself is a positive step towards assimilation or accomodation as it is an open field, unfenced by preconceptions and limiting beliefs for labor. New concepts are able to be explored in the process of such disorientation.

Let us examine the case of a woman who maintains the belief that pain is oppressive, weakening, and humiliating. Intellectually, she may have even decided that pain in birth was "different," yet she has not had the opportunity to test this

---

*According to Piaget, assimilation occurs when new concepts are fit into an individual's already existing cognitive structure. Accomodation occurs when the cognitive structure must change in order to accept the new concept.

decision emotionally. As a therapist, I have often witnessed the necessity for intellectual insight to become emotional experience if change in behavior, attitude, and quality of life is to occur. As the woman experiences the sounds of pain in labor, she is confronted with her own emotional beliefs and reactions to labor prior to the actual labor process. She has time to panic now, to admit her fear, to become disoriented, and to re-learn her belief about pain as it relates to labor. She can explore her reactions and discover her own beliefs about labor before, rather than during her labor.

Such a woman might find her old beliefs surfacing, and experience dissonance with the reactions of the teacher as the role model. Such a state of dissonance is a highly charged energy state, and also a very vulnerable one. It is a state in which the woman may no longer believe fully in her old beliefs as they become challenged by the teacher/therapist, yet has not fully developed new beliefs from which she can organize her perceptions of her childbirth experience to be consonant with the teacher/therapist. This kind of situation can facilitate a quicksand effect, where survival mechanisms are mobilized psycho-emotionally. The result is an intense focus on learning, or re-learning a new attitude.

Through explanation of fears and feelings about the tape, the woman, often with support of other group members, can move through her state of dissonance, towards assimilation or accomodation of new learning to an eventual state of consonance in herself. At this point a woman has plenty of time for such a transformation. Her birth is imminent within the next six weeks, which adds to her urgency of focus in the classes, yet she is able to consolidate her new awareness in the next month of classes. She has the time and the motivation to explore her emotions. Giving class members permission to talk about a full range of emotional responses to the tape is an important impetus for developing self-awareness.

The teacher as role model for the concept of "healthy" pain continues. Her matter-of-fact acceptance of the audio-tape, verification of the sound as expression of pain, and answering of questions about the labor on tape presents to the class members the resiliency of the body in labor. In the context of childbirth, pain does not weaken a woman. The teacher's positive attitude towards the pain is the stability that the members of the class respond to emotionally, learning the attitude of the teacher herself. Previously, fear of such pain may have been learned through a mother, a grandmother, a sister, or other cultural role models in much the same manner. It is of utmost importance to be aware of the power of the teacher as a vehicle for re-learning. Such role modeling is in itself a form of indirect hypnosis, or suggestion, not to be underestimated especially following the emotional experience of the audio-tape. It is imperative that the teacher be confident and genuine in her responses and in her attitude towards birth as both healthy and painful. It is necessary, therefore, that the teacher herself has worked through fear of pain, and has been able to accept it as a part of a unique, beautiful, and powerful experience. She will then be able to deal with fears of pain truthfully and positively. *The depth and richness of the labor experience is communicated simultaneously with the acceptance of pain.* This is a form of conditioning, whereby the beauty and meaning of birth is associated with the pain as a part of the meaningfulness of birth. Therefore, the mechanics of labor are fused with the emotional significance of the experience. As a woman experiences pain in labor, she does not need to fight it as a negative or degrading experience. She can accept the beauty of birth to include pain, working in body and mind towards the emergence of her child into the world. She is in harmony with herself.

After time has been allowed for expression of feeling, another part of the tape is played in which the last twenty minutes or half hour of the labor is experienced through sound, and the completion of the labor as the baby is born is heard. The audio-tape continues after birth, and the joy, excitement and tenderness of the experience is often tearfully shared by the class members.

The birth experience shared by the family on tape is easily identified with, reminding class members of their own intimacy with others. The tears of acceptance that so often flow from class members include the reality of pain as part of the experience of labor and birth. The beginnings of the belief in pain as healthy have been planted in the psyche.

Class members are encouraged to think about the audio-tape over the course of the week before their next class, and to let their emotions surface as they do so, exploring issues which they may then bring back to the following class.

The above process is described as it takes place in general. However, let us consider the effect of this second class on a woman, perhaps a single mother, ambivalent about becoming a mother. Whatever she fears, whatever conflict may be present, the power of the sounds of labor and birth brings her to an inner reflection and contemplation of who she is and how she will prepare herself to handle her own labor experience. For each woman, an inner exploration of fears begins. The single mother may be at a loss for being without a partner or feeling unable to care for her baby by herself once it is born. Whatever the ambivalence, conflicts that need to be resolved will surface. The fact that she does not have the father of the child with her to share in the birth is a reality in her preparation. If, in fact, it is a sensitive area for her, her feelings of loneliness or resentment as she sees pregnant women with partners in stores, in the medical setting, and in classes, is a measure of the degree to which she is in conflict over her present situation. It can be an opportunity for growth to address this issue and to help her resolve it. Here again, the teacher/therapist will serve as a role model in feeling comfortable with the woman's discomfort due to conflict. Encouraging her towards resolution through confrontation with reality and conveying an attitude of acceptance for the emotional pain she will need to work through is of great importance. The teacher/therapist needs to be able to recognize and facilitate individual work as necessary, and to be able to serve the best interests of her clients by not trying to avoid painful issues, but rather by conveying acceptance of emotional pain, just as she conveys acceptance of the physical pain dealt with in the class. If she is able to do this, the seeds of self-illumination and acceptance can take root, so that the pregnant woman may be facilitated in resolving crucial issues in her life. Again the significance of the childbirth experience on the woman's self-esteem and confidence in mothering deserves being repeated. The first purpose of the audio-tape has been accomplished when conflict surfaces and self-exploration ensues. The nature of the self-exploration is individual for each person.

Elements of the Audio-tape

When choosing a tape to use in preparing women for childbirth, it is important that the labor and delivery be a totally normal one in which no physical or psychological interventions were needed. Women are being taught a normal delivery. It should be a labor in which the woman was uninhibited in making sound so that the vocalization is coming from a natural deep breathing, developing into an expression of pain as labor progresses. Power, strength, and pain will be predominant rather than fear and apprehension.

Class members are assured that women birth individually and that vocalization is by no means mandatory for a natural birth. However, the fact that most women given permission for spontaneity, do in fact vocalize during contractions is significant. As a woman yells, she may automatically breathe deeply down to the diaphragm. The diaphragm expands when it is engaged in making sound. Because of its placement (right above the uterus in a pregnant woman) such expansion often exerts force for pushing the baby out.

Women should never be pressured into making sound in labor. They are granted their individual manner of giving birth and are encouraged to make sound should it feel right in labor.

Most women vocalize to some extent if they are not conditioned to be quiet in labor in their childbirth preparation. Traditionally, to be "in control" and to be quiet have been synonymous in the hosptial setting, and often at home as well. However, often a woman needs to "let go" with sound in order to be truly "in control" or "at one" with her body process. Vocalization can take the form of dispersal of energy which is not conducive to labor, in which case coaching a woman to remain quiet to focus her attention and energy on the inside of her body may be necessary. However, due to cultural conditioning, it is much easier to coach a woman to be quiet, if in fact vocalization is dispersing rather than focusing her energy, than to coach a woman to let go through vocalization, if in fact she needs to. In classes, women usually respond positively to such matter-of-fact information, and become increasingly comfortable with letting go and loosening inhibitions during labor. Much of their confidence and comfort with doing so lies in the fact that their labor attendants are accepting of their expressions of pain in labor. They do not need to protect others from the intensity of the experience.

The sound of the audio-tape of labor represents what a contraction feels like on the inside, whether or not such feeling is expressed vocally. Permission to vocalize is an indirect hypnotic message that pain in labor is normal. The purpose of the audio-tape is twofold. First it serves to bring conflict to the surface and facilitate personal growth, emphasizing the opportunity for learning and mind-body integration. Secondly, it augments realistic preparation which decreases the possibility of mind-body dissonance in labor.

The following relaxation exercise is given immediately following discussion of the birth audio-tape. Because of the intensity of experience of the tape, the relaxation exercise is usually participated in with great attentiveness and sincerity. Class members may be very vulnerable and emotionally open at this time, rendering them at an optimal focus for learning. The audio-tape experience emphasizes the purpose of the material being presented. Class members therefore tend to be filled with a sense of purpose and direction, exactly the psycho-emotional state needed for labor and birth. Women are being guided towards the frame of mind most conducive to the kind of delivery they have expressed the desire for, i.e., a meaningful experience in which they prepare for cooperation with natural forces.

Relaxation Exercise

Pregnant women are instructed to lie down comfortably on the floor, their partners sitting or lying beside them. A relaxation induction is given for both men and women in which they relax each part of the body through direction of breath. Deep breathing that has been practiced from the first class is incorporated as a means of releasing tension and deepening relaxation in each part of the body.

When the relaxation induction is completed, the husband or labor partner is instructed to open his/her eyes and to become attentive to his/her partner. The partner is asked to check the woman's body both visually and by touch for full relaxation. Places that are observed to be tense are worked on with verbal feedback and coaching going on between the woman and her labor support person. Partners sequentially lift each limb of their woman's body off the floor a couple of inches, testing for limpness and lack of tension, as they release the limb.

After tense areas of the body have been identified, the women have a sense of how they can continue to practice relaxation throughout the next week. Body awareness has been heightened, and particular areas of stress recognized. Areas of the body in which tension is held can be relaxed through deep breathing at any time during the day.

Women are then instructed to tense one leg as they hold it a few inches off the ground for one or two minutes, while keeping the rest of the body loose and relaxed. Their partners check the rest of the body (opposite leg particularly) to make sure that the tension in the tensed leg is not transferred to any other part of the body. This process deepens body awareness further and facilitates conscious control of each part of the body to respond to the directive to relax.

The process is repeated, tensing only one arm, working to isolate the tension in that arm without responding with tenseness in the rest of the body. Twice more it is repeated, tensing the right arm and left leg (crossing over tension in both sides of the body, without letting such tension move to the left arm and right leg) and then tensing the right arm and left leg, working to isolate tension in these two areas of the body only, relaxing all other parts.

This last part of the exercise (tensing opposite arm and leg) is particularly useful in discovering how much conscious control is available for relaxation and to what extent a woman needs to work on her ability to relax.

Relaxation of the total body at one time is the easiest task to acquire and the first to be mastered. However, once such relaxation is achieved, it is necessary to heighten awareness and conscious control of the relaxation process. This exercise serves the purpose of further educating the woman to her ability to gain control through her body. During labor, a woman's uterus is contracting very firmly. The uterus is tense, hard, and meant to be so during a contraction. During contractions it is important for the woman to not respond to the tenseness in one part of her body (the uterus) by transferring tension into other parts of the body. She will need to learn such ability to direct and focus her energy for relaxation in order not to automatically respond by tensing the rest of her body. This exercise usually brings women to an awareness of the importance of relaxation. It also motivates them to practice relaxation, incorporating it into their life style. If a woman is able to respond to contractions by relaxing, she is using less of her available energy for the work of each contraction. Relaxation also renders the contractions more successful at bringing the baby down, if in fact the baby's head is not being met by tight vaginal walls of muscular resistance. Pain, in general, is automatically responded to with resistance and tension. Therefore, it is necessary for a woman to practice the exercises in order to learn a healthier response to pain in labor.

Yells, or sounds of pain can help to release tension from the body. Relaxation does not mean silence. On the contrary, a woman can experience greater relaxation through expressive adaptation. Vocalization is a common vehicle for creative adaptation in labor. Vocalization during contractions can stimulate total relaxation in between contractions. It is in the time between contractions that a woman can drift, sometimes into the heightened or altered states of consciousness that have been documented by women in labor.[4] On the labor audio-tape used for teaching, the quality of sound, usually quiet or non-existent between contractions, is very definite, marking the beginning and end of a contraction.

Women return home to incorporate the experience of the second class, encompassing in themselves the intimacy of their own bodies with the natural forces of the universe.

REFERENCES

1. LeBoyer, F. *Birth Without Violence.* New York, Knopf, 1975.

2. Bandura, A. *Principles of Behavior Modification.* San Francisco, Holt, Reinhart, & Winston, 1968 and Gellhorn, E. *Behavioral Analysis of Drug Action.* New York, Appleton, Century, Crofts, 1968.

3. Maternity Association, *Birth Atlas,* New York, 6th edition, 1975.

4. Lang, R. *The Birth Book.* Felton, New Genesis Press, 1977.

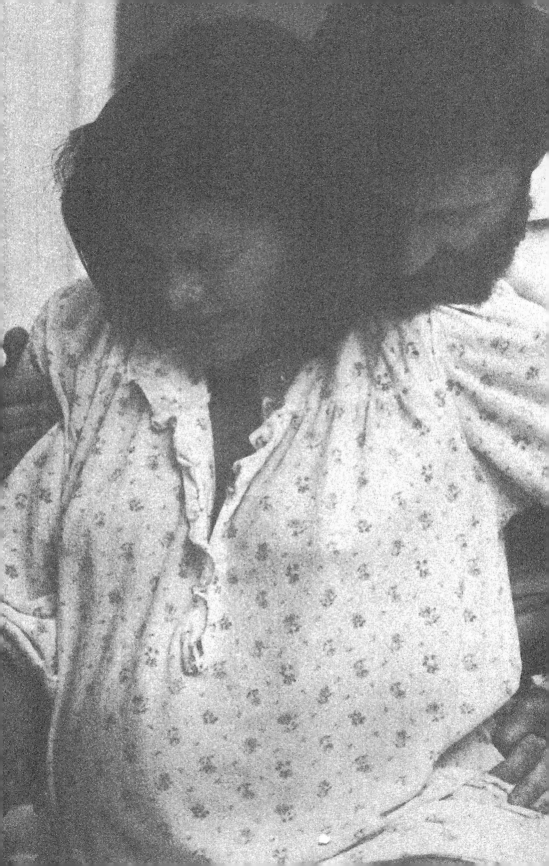

Chapter Six

Psychophysiological Integration

LABOR AND BIRTH are taught as a continuously unfolding process that grows out of pregnancy. Stages of labor are referred to only if women have questions about them from various books. Phases of labor is a more appropriate term and may be used in lieu of "stages," as "phases" imply a "travelling through" rather than something that is set or "staged," and static. An association may also be made for a woman with performance anxiety about birth, as a "stage" is also a place for theatrical performance. However, it is questionable whether either of these terms is needed for description of labor, as both tend to artificially divide a whole into parts.

In classes, women are introduced to labor as a phenomenon which begins with early labor, which may go on for days or weeks. Early labor is generally considered as 1-4 cms. dilation for a first baby and 1-5 or 6 for a subsequent baby. Women are encouraged to go about their daily lives, with some adjustment or relaxation, but to do all their normal activities in between contractions, letting the contractions come and go, centering attention on the contraction as it comes and returning to daily activity as it wanes.

Labor gradually grows more and more painful, creating an increasingly intense focus. When a woman can no longer go about her daily activities in between contractions, she is considered to be in hard labor, focusing all of her energy between and during contractions on her body giving birth. It is during this later phase of labor that women are encouraged to vocalize as needed or desired.

The phenomenon of "transition" is not described in classes, as it has not been my experience that such a phenomenon exists. If women are not taught to expect a period of panic, nausea, and unexpected changes in perception which are labelled "transition",* they ordinarily do not experience it. As a woman expects her labor to increase in intensity until the baby is born, she normally travels through the said "transition" period, in a continuous manner to her initial style of coping. Description of transition is an artificially divided piece of labor as described in childbirth literature.

One of the greatest dangers of the myth of "transition" is the proclamation by well-meaning childbirth teachers that it is the hardest time, and from there on it is easy. Women of first babies are led to believe that it will not hurt to push (second phase) and that it will even feel good and be easy.

Many a first mother is mentally ready to quit when she finds it is not true for her, since she had not prepared herself for pain or hard labor beyond this point. This delusion has caused many arrests in this part of labor, and is not realistic preparation.

Pushing during labor is taught as something which may or may not happen without conscious effort. A woman may feel as if her uterus is doing all the work, while she rides through the contraction. Or she may experience a need to consciously exert the effort of pushing deliberately in order to birth her baby. An outgrowth of vocalization is often a natural bearing down, or pushing sound, which can help to expand the diaphragm, creating a pressure on the top of the uterus, helping to push the baby out.

To help stimulate a lack of inhibition about sound and to simulate the effect of the pressure of a contraction and the releasing energy of sound, the following exercise is done in class.

Sound Release

Class members are instructed to take a deep breath and to hold the breath and begin to bear down, (pushing as if going to the bathroom). Holding the breath and pushing simulates the pressure of a contraction building. When there is a sign of increased pressure, and class members are working hard, instructions are given to very suddenly open the throat, to release constriction of the throat completely. If the exercise is done correctly, the person doing the exercise will spontaneously emit a very open sound. The greater the inner build of pressure, the greater and longer the sound. This exercise usually needs to be

---

*Transition is described as a "panicky" time, one in which the woman will experience confusion, nausea and loss of control.

done several times before a person will permit themselves the lack of inhibition necessary to experience it. Women are also encouraged to use the natural body function of moving their bowels in order to experience the difference in quality between holding their breath and pushing feces out, and opening their throat and using sound to help to push.

During a contraction, the pressure is many times the intensity of such an exercise and is readily apparent, so that the open throat can be an immediate response. As a woman emits sound, her pushing will come from the diaphragm, pushing down on the uterus (i.e. effective pushing as opposed to ineffectively pushing with the stomach or thighs). It is this combination of letting go, while pushing, that can create the easiest and least resistant passageway for the baby's descent.

The baby's descent (or second phase of labor) is referred to as a period in which a change in quality of experience will evolve as the baby moves out of the womb and into the vagina. Women are prepared to expect it to be a very "active" time, as opposed to the more "passive" yielding state that can take place during first phase of labor. Pushing the baby out is a period of active yielding, and needs to be respected as such.

The energy of birth is an aggressive force. It takes enormous energy to create and move a human body from the plane of non-physical existence (prior to conception) to emerge into the plane of physical experience (birth). It is important that a woman not be afraid of aggression in this context, as it is a healthy aggression like the turbulence of rainstorms, the barrelling of thunder clouds as they clap together. Again, the belief in a "gentle" birth cannot preclude this aggressive thrust of life, without the possible side effects of psychophysiological dissonance in labor.

With the terrible beauty of the thunderstorm comes the quiet, the gentle, the stillness of fresh wet grass under opened sky. The gentleness in nature is a response to the aggressive beauty and yielding of the earth.

As a woman learns to weave aggression into her natural and culturally conditioned gentleness, she releases herself from the restrictive role of the feminine in our society. She liberates herself to the strength and power found in tenderness. Giving birth can be one way for a woman to reveal to herself her individual tapestry. It is not the only way. It is simply one of nature's gifts of self-discovery.

At birth, self-discovery has just begun, and the workings of the maternal-infant relationship trace the deserts, forest floors, and rivers of a woman's heart. If she has begun the journey in a positive manner, she has that much fortune of a good beginning.

Slides of Labor and Birth

When choosing slides to show in classes, I attempt to compile sets of slides that distill the emotional counterparts of aggression, beauty, and gentleness in the experience. Slides of pained expressions, yelling mouths, and silent smiles are all necessary for a realistic portrayal of labor and birth.

During the third class, three sets of slides of births are shown, while ideally the birth attendants present at these deliveries speak about her/his role in each experience. Throughout the narrative the birth attendant (either physician or midwife) if possible (and, if not, the teacher/therapist) can give natural hypnotic suggestion for normal delivery. As attention to the slides is a primary focus, the opportunity for hypnotic effect is present. The visual sense is totally occupied, creating the kind of trance state familiar to movie and television viewers who are unwilling to tear their gaze from the screen for any other environmental stimulus. In a story-telling voice, and using emphasis, phrasing, and the voice dynamics mentioned in Chapter IV, the birth attendant is able to describe each normal delivery, emphasizing the natural healthy process as it evolves, emphasizing a normal third phase of labor* and the bonding experience that follows.

Class members are able to ask questions during this time, and all questions are answered with the incorporation of a healthy delivery included in the response. The manner in which this is done is so varied that it cannot be described here. In the unusual case of a woman being totally absorbed in the possibility of complication, the woman is invited to explore her questions in depth in an individual appointment, so that the class retains its healthful orientation. Questions about complication are answered in such a way as to *not* hypnotically introduce fear or suggestion for complication in a woman while she is in a type of trance state.

It is important to keep the class on a general level of healthful expectation for labor and delivery. Maintaining a focus on normal delivery can be achieved even while answering questions about complication, if the needs of the questioner are not such that the attention of the class as a whole becomes focused mostly on these

---

*The third stage or phase of labor is the expulsion of the placenta.

possibilities. An approach to prenatal care is achieved whereby all questions regarding complication *can be answered,* but such questions generally take place *outside classes.* The significance of this shift is that as a couple defines themselves as coming to classes to learn to prepare for their delivery, it is necessary that the learning focus (which is a hypnotic one) be expectation for normal labor and delivery. In this manner, the pregnant woman does not identify with the details of Cesarean section in a setting which is provided for preparation for normal birth. Identification is a powerful form of learning and not to be underestimated in the classroom setting. In the educational setting description of complication becomes preparation for complication for the pregnant woman. This preparation may become an expectation for the abnormal, precluding the ability to acquire healthy attitudes for normal delivery.

Too often, extensive discussion of complication takes place in one or more classes in a childbirth preparation course which negates the previously taught normalcy of birth. The emotionality of fear and group participation in the visualization of each complication as it is discussed may facilitate an identification and interfere with healthy delivery. This kind of negative identification can become a belief the woman has about herself in labor. It may also serve as a self-fulfilling prophecy, if the woman is already predisposed to complication due to acculturation or personal background. (An example of such a predisposition for complication might be a woman whose grandmother hemorrhaged in birth, and who believes herself to be very much like her grandmother.)

Classes may be a way of re-learning a woman's approach to birth, and the class setting needs to be respected for its influence on expectations and beliefs. To focus on complication in the class environment is to teach complication, since for the pregnant woman, all that is being said is taken on a very personal level. As labor is described, a woman imagines herself in labor, wonders about herself, her possible reactions. When pushing is talked about, a woman imagines herself pushing. This intimate level of participation takes place spontaneously because of the pregnancy which is the motivation for the classes. There would not exist so strong an influence in a classroom setting of nurses, doctors, childbirth educators, who were discussing complications on a more objective level, because of the absence of immediate identification. However, the medical professionals also suffer from an intense focus on the abnormal. This focus may be limiting to the extent that it obstructs the ability to visualize, imagine, or recognize the healthy process as it occurs.[1]

Because of the imminency of birth to each woman in the childbirth classes, information can be absorbed on a very intimate level. It is this level of intimacy that needs to be respected in classes, so that the learning or re-learning of beliefs through identification can take place in such a way that directs a woman towards normal delivery. Discussion of complications can take place outside of the hypnotic environment of the classes.

The slides that are chosen to be shown in classes must also be recognized as imparting significant learning to the class members. As in a movie, identification with the heroine takes place. Slides of excessive bleeding, or other complications, are not beneficial. Normal delivery, in a variety of styles, positions, and settings is the message of the slide presentations.

Touch Relaxation and Focus for Yielding

Either before or after the slide presentation in the third class, couples are instructed in participation of a form of relaxation which requires no verbal communication, but only the communication of touch.

The pregnant woman lies comfortably, focusing her attention on the sensation of her partner's touch. She concentrates on yielding, responding to the touch of her partner's fingers and hands on each part of her body by relaxing each area as he touches her (legs, arms, torso, pelvis, neck, etc.). Her partner pays attention to areas of tension with which they have both become familiar with in her body during the past three weeks of classes. Gentle touching and massaging of these areas is done to loosen any remaining tightness.

There is no talking between partners, as it is an exercise in communication through touch communicating to the body to relax, to let go. Generally a feeling of peace and calm fills the room as the women become relaxed, yielding to the touch and love of their partners.

After the relaxation seems complete, the partners are instructed in the application of pressure (increasing to pain) to a part of the woman's body (usually behind her knee) which builds slowly. This growing pressure is a weak simulation for a contraction. Women are instructed to begin using deep breathing, or even a gentle moaning in order to yield to the pressure-pain as it builds, as opposed to fighting the pain with a wall of tension. This yielding response to pain can be learned and is often used by long distance runners as they come up against the "wall."* It commonly takes at least 3-4 attempts at applying pressure-pain before the partners of the pregnant women are effective. The woman deserves the opportunity of this challenge, and finds herself understanding the use of deep breathing and sound as a form of concentration and facilitation of yielding to each contraction. This exercise, although not nearly the quality of sensation of a contraction, does simulate the quality of focus, or hypnotic trance state described in Chapter IV. It is this quality of focus for yielding to the contraction that is the most valuable tool for childbirth preparation. Through application of this quality of focus, or relaxed concentration, a woman is less likely to fight contractions.

Class members are encouraged to practice this exercise at home, again with the emphasis of responsibility for their preparation on themselves.

---

*The "wall" is described to be a painful point when the long distance runner feels like stopping, however by continuing, the runner breaks through the "wall."

REFERENCES

1. Illich, I. *Medical Nemesis*. New York, Pantheon Press, 1976.

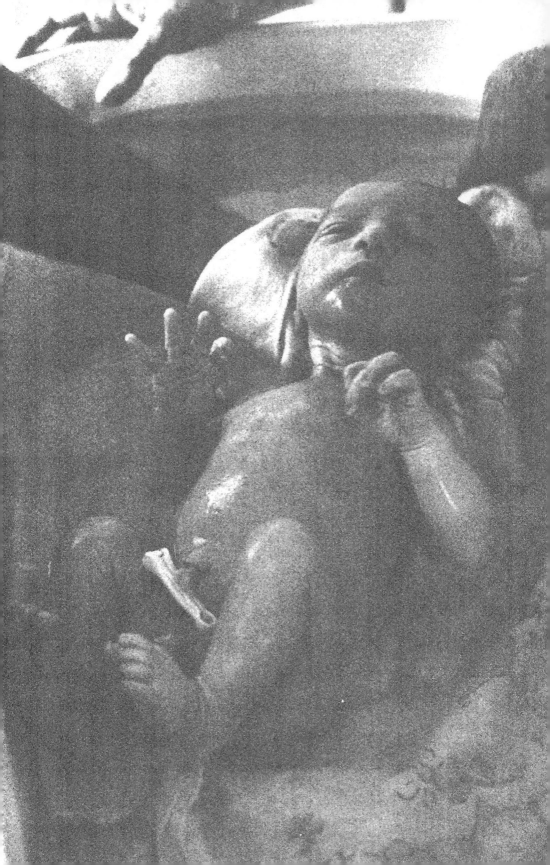

Chapter Seven

The Newborn

THE FOURTH CLASS is the only class in the series that focuses exclusively on the newborn and what happens after the birth. This is because the support and information are already part of the birthing services in a holistic framework, which should include 2-3 home visits during the three days after birth and subsequent follow-up at one week to one month postpartum. Adjustment can be made according to the needs of each setting into which this material is being used. It is during close contact with families after birth that difficulties with nursing, sibling rivalry, and other postpartum issues can be addressed. Postpartum visits are an important element of a Holistic Prenatal Care program. Within a holistic health setting, the main focus of childbirth classes can be birth. This focus is appropriate and enjoyable to the pregnant woman.

During the fourth class of the late series discussion of the presence of colostrum, changes in milk production as the baby grows,[1] and nutritional information for nursing mothers and babies is covered. Supplemental feedings for the working mother are usually discussed on an individual basis during the course of prenatal and postpartum care. Questions about breastfeeding are often answered by other mothers in the class. Breastfeeding is a good subject for group sharing and discussion which could be the beginnings of a support group for parents after their babies are born.

The general appearance of the newborn at birth and in the first month of life, is also a point of discussion in this class. Again, class members may be able to share prior experience with one another. Certain characteristics of the newborn are recognized including molding of the head, vernix, baby acne, properties and care of the umbilical cord, and the bonding phenomenon. Care of the newborn is discussed and changes of life-style in parenthood may also be recognized, as in the series of early classes. The most controversial of issues, circumcision, is discussed last in the fourth class.

The purpose of the discussion on circumcision is to educate people to the difference between the religious and cultural myths about the need for circumcision and the medical facts. Through education and discussion of feelings, parents can become aware of the difference between personal values and factual information. There is never an emphasis on right or wrong regarding circumcision, and it is important that the childbirth educator recognize and respect the decision of the parents. It is not the role of the childbirth educator to judge, or to recommend, but rather to demystify the reasons for the process of circumcision in order for parents to make an educated decision.

Circumcision is introduced and defined as a surgical procedure. Like any other surgical procedure, circumcision carries with it risk of complication. The procedure itself is described realistically. The need to strap the infant down to avoid sudden moves which might cause error in the circumcision is explained. The fact that circumcision is painful is verified by those mothers who have been present, as well as nurses and other medical people. To mislead parents by telling then that it does not "hurt" the baby any more than a PKU test,* in which the baby's heel is pricked, or using some other mild analogy is not only unkind, but unprofessional. This kind of misrepresentation so common in the medical profession, does not prepare a mother for the screams of a baby in pain and may cause her regret. This is particularly true if, in fact, the misrepresentation accounted for a large part of her decision in the first place.

The Jewish ceremony of circumcision allows the mother to hold the infant as the operation occurs.

Complication of circumcision occurs at a rate of six cases out of every 1,000. The most common complication is the need to return for further surgery during infancy or later in childhood to remove small skin attachments that remain when the foreskin does not tear cleanly from the penis. Returning for completion of the circumcision at a later time is necessary in this case to avoid ripping into the penis. The latter is another complication which is

---

*PKU test is a test for phenylketonuria involving a small needle prick in the baby's heel.

recognized. A complication rate of 6 out of 1,000 is low, yet does exist. This rate of complication is significant as it represents pathology that is created during the course of a medically non-indicated surgical operation.

Scar tissue resulting from circumcision which may be particularly thick may cause complications later in life affecting the ability to maintain an erection without pain. This may be due to the scar tissue being not as stretchable as the regular skin tissue.

More serious but highly rare complications (one out of every 20,000 cases) have included bleeding to death and cutting into the penis to such a degree that partial castration takes place (usually due to malfunction of hospital equipment). This last complication is very unlikely to occur, yet is mentioned in light of the fact the circumcision is a surgical procedure with no medical reason for performance. All surgery carries some risk. Parents learn about the procedure of circumcision and possible complications. After information has been presented, myths concerning the "medical need' for circumcision are discussed. These include the myth of cleanliness and the myth that being uncircumcised causes cancer.

The Myth of Cleanliness

Cleanliness has been linked with "next to Godliness" by many religions. The roots of circumcision are indeed religious, and it is not the religious reasons for circumcision that are addressed, for these are outside of the area of medical judgement. Rather it is the myth of cleanliness often perpetuated through religion that is demystified. Interpreters of religion have always had a difficult time integrating sexuality and sensuality as healthy aspects of life experience. The cultural counterpart of this belief that sex/sensuality is unhealthy is the commonplace belief that "sex is dirty". Worse is the belief that sex and violence are closely linked. The last association is evident in magazine advertisements[2] in which alcohol or cigarettes may be advertised commonly with the body of a woman in the foreground. The image of a dagger or gun is embedded in the background, not readily apparent to the naked eye, but easily identified with a magnifying glass.*

---

*The result may be an unconscious association of a woman's body (sex) with the gun or dagger (violence) in the background. This association is used by the advertisement industry to sell products, as it appeals to sexual and violent urges simultaneously, and subliminally. The manufacturer counts on this association to sell the product.

The premise of cleanliness for advocation of circumcision is religiously and culturally rooted in a distortion of sexuality. Cleanliness bears no relation to circumcision, given the normal attention to bathing present in this culture. Mothers have often been informed by well-meaning pediatricians that if their baby is not to be circumcised that they must take special care to regularly retract the foreskin and wash the penis in order to avoid infection. When infection occurs due to irritation of the foreskin by prematurely stretching it through such early retraction, the mother believes she has not washed it diligently enough. The fact is that the foreskin is present to protect the penis from infection. The foreskin cannot be pulled back on a newborn without considerable effort and stretching of the skin tissues. This is for a good reason, as it is not meant to be pulled back, but keeps the penis sterile during the first year of life without need of scrupulous scrubbing. Pulling back the foreskin produces irritation and can introduce infection. By the end of one year, the foreskin has usually become gradually looser naturally and can be retracted very easily. At this point, washing the penis beneath the foreskin becomes an ordinary part of hygiene, and continues, just as a woman washes her labia and vaginal opening. Without premature retraction, incidence of infections of the penis are rare. Given a natural orientation towards touching and washing the penis, a growing boy need not fear infection due to not being circumcised. The myth of cleanliness as a reason for circumcision implies that the penis itself is a dirty part of the body which cannot be cleaned as any other area of the body. It is as if the penis suffers from an association with sex.

The Cancer Myth

The second myth addressed arises out of a study by Dagher.[3] The study stated that the rate of cancer found in men who were not circumcised and their wives was significantly greater when compared to circumcised men. The fallacy in this study lies in the fact that only men already having penile cancer were studied. When a similar, but much larger study was done in Sweden, with uncircumcised men, there was a significantly lower incidence of cancer.[4] In another study in India, Moslem women whose husbands were circumcised were compared to a group of Parsee women whose husbands were uncircumcised. The Parsee women had less cervical cancer as well as better hygiene.[5] There was found to be no correlation between lack of circumcision and penile or cervical cancer. The most common theme underlying all of these studies was multiple sexual partners, high incidence of venereal disease and poor hygiene which was associated with higher levels of penile and cervical cancer. The precipitating factor for cancer was not circumcision.

Having demystified the two medical myths about circumcision, there are other issues which need to be introduced. These include the psychological reasons for circumcision, such as a boy wanting circumcision when he is older and an uncircumcised boy's fears of not fitting into a family in which the father and/or brothers are circumcised. This concern may also extend to peers and schoolmates as the boy grows up.

It is necessary to facilitate discussion about these concerns and provide information about how families have dealt with differences in circumcised and uncircumcised members. Simple case examples, such as one man who was not circumcised due to a low Apgar* score at birth can be illuminating. His response to being uncircumcised in his family was that it was one of the many "differences" between himself and his brothers.

Another mother who had decided not to circumcise her baby due to a bad experience with her first son's circumcision which needed to be re-done three times, explained to her ten-year-old son that she did not know as much ten years ago as she did now, and that she would not have chosen to circumcise him if she had it to do over. She broke the false belief that mothers cannot make mistakes or change over time.

The question of whether circumcision at a later age is more painful or complicated can be answered with the following factual information. Newborns are not given any anesthesia for pain during circumcision due to the risk of complications. The foreskin itself is very tight and unretractable, therefore potential of complication is greater in the newborn than in a man, or an older boy. By one year of age the foreskin can usually be retracted easily, therefore potential for complications may be less by this age. Men and older boys can also be given anesthesia for the operation, alleviating the physical pain of the operation itself.

Further facilitation of discussion of the changing times is also necessary for the mother or father who would decide to circumcise due to a belief that all their son's peers will be circumcised in the future. This is a changing situation, as more parents are deciding not to circumcise, especially with the American Academy of

---

*The Apgar score is a point system used to evaluate the condition of the baby at birth.

Pediatrics withdrawal of support for circumcision.[6] Also, it should be made clear that the circumcised child has no choice as he grows older into manhood, while the uncircumcised child does have the ability to participate in the decision should he consider circumcision as he grows into adulthood. Often there is present in the class a man who exercised the option of circumcision in adulthood due to army stipulations who may share his experience of it as an adult. Circumcision is presented realistically, as an irreversible operation.

It is the responsibility of the childbirth educator to demystify circumcision and to offer pertinent information so that parents can exercise their own judgment. It is important that personal values, such as religious reasons for circumcision, are separated from the myths in order for responsible decisions to be made and for parents to feel resolved about their decisions. I have heard many mothers express regret about their past decision to circumcise when they become cognizant of the "facts" they had based their decision on were actually just assumptions, or cultural myths. This can be avoided by accurately addressing the psychological and medical issues involved prior to circumcison.

The childbirth educator is most effective in a supportive rather than judgemental role, providing a framework in which parents can explore their feelings, reactions, reasons and values regarding circumcision. The importance of tradition as a reason for circumcision and traditional religion, most commonly present in the Jewish culture, lies in individual values and can be supported appropriately. The significance of the information provided is the stimulation for women and men to identify their own values and to accept clearly their decisions made within their own personal value system. Through this type of process, women and men are able to distinguish between what are personal values and what is factual information.

In many cases, parents take the next few weeks to contemplate their decision, and may even wait until the child is born to actually decide. There is no rush as circumcision can take place at any time in life.

REFERENCES

1. Pryor, K. *Nursing Your Baby*. New York, Harper and Row, 1963.

2. Gerbner, G. and Gross, L. The Scary World of TV's Heavy Viewer. *Psychol. Today*, April, 1976, p. 41; Peterson, B., et al. Television Advertising and Drug Use. *Am. J. Public Health* 66 (10): 975-978, 1976.; Singer, J.L. and Singer, D.J. Television: A Member of the Family. *Yale Review*, 1977; Feingold, M. and Johnson, G.T. Television Violence. *New Eng. J. Med.* 296: 424-427, 1977.

3. Dagher, R. Carcinoma of the Penis and the Anti-circumcision Crusade. *Journal of Urology*, Aug. 1970, pp. 291-297; Hardner, G. J. Carcinoma of the Penis: Analysis of Therapy in 100 Consecutive Cases. *Journal of Urology*, 108:428-429, Sept. 1972.

4. Acta, P. Circumcision and Prostate Cancer. *acta Med. Scand.* 178:493-504, 1965. Hanash, K. A. Carcinoma of the Penis: A Clinical Pathological Study. *J. Urol.* Aug. 291-297, 1970.

5. Aitken-Swan, J. and Baird, D. Circumcision and Cancer of the Cervix. *Brit. J. Cancer*, 6: 881-886, 1950; Terris, N. Relation of Circumcision to Cancer of the Cervix. *Am. J. Ob. Gyn.* 117: 1056-1066, Dec. 1973.

6. Committee on Fetus and Newborn: Report of the Ad Hoc Task Force on Circumcision. *Peds.* 56:610, 1975.

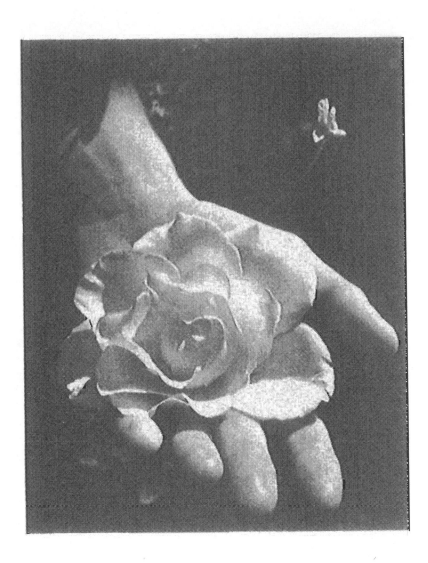

Chapter Eight

The Catalyst for Personal Growth: Self Confidence

IN THIS CLASS, a set of detailed slides of a birth are shown. There are usually not many questions at this point, but rather a sense of completion and an air of confidence in the process. Again, it is important that the slides of the birth show a normal delivery, and one in which the woman's individuality is also apparent. This gives a woman permission for her own personality to be expressed in labor, and for her own individuality to be validated. Roles of other family members are apparent in the set of slides I usually use which includes a brother, husband, and two daughters in the labor and birth sequence.* Individual work is indicated if anxiety persists at high levels for any class member.

Included in the last class is another audio-tape of the last 30 minutes of a normal labor and birth. Again, intensity of labor contractions is measured through vocalization. The response to this second audio-tape is usually one of relaxed acceptance. The sounds of expression of pain have been integrated into a healthy acceptance of pain in labor and the depth and beauty of the experience is the major effect on class members. The half hour of continuous laboring on the audio-tape takes a woman through the experience vicariously. The quality of this experience of simply following the last half hour of an actual labor and birth by ear usually stimulates the yielding attitude necessary for birth. The emotional response to the birth on the audio-tape is of the same quality as the attitude of yielding to the unknown, revealing and vulnerable.

It is at this class that other members of the family are invited who might be present at the birth—sibling, friends, relatives. It is an opportunity for each of them to explore his or her own attitudes and feelings about labor and birth and to facilitate final

---

*Dania's Birth, by Suzanne Arms, available from Suzanne Arms Productions, 151 Lytton Ave., Palo Alto, California 94304.

organization of the support system for the laboring woman. Assimilation of the newborn into the family is easiest when each member participates in the birth experience through being present during labor and birth, aiding in preparation, or by helping afterwards. This is a time for siblings to familiarize themselves with labor sounds and to ask questions that have not been answered. The slides also encourage children to identify with the experience, as two siblings are present in the slides shown.

No new information is presented at this time, as the last class serves as a final emotional completion of the preparation. Through classes, a woman has been guided inwards to identify her own strength and has been introduced to a deeper potential for yielding than she has probably ever experienced before. She is dealing more intimately with nature through her pregnancy. Her two major resources are her own strength and her ability to yield, to let go of expectations, so that adjustment to the labor process can take place in her own creative style. Confidence influences the journey through labor by increasing endurance and strength; it is the attitude of yielding, however, that allows for adjustment necessary to an unknown situation.

By the last class, a woman has usually integrated the concept of healthy pain in labor, and is looking forward to the learning experience of labor and birth. Pregnancy has brought her to a place of completion, of fullness and of yielding. Fears and anxieties have been addressed, expressed, and worked through to the place of acceptance of the unknown journey ahead. Plans and preparations are completed and now is the time to forget them, to let go of expectations. To know the preparation is thorough and complete is her base of strength. To forget about her plans and expectations and to trust to the unknown is her source of yielding, an attitude of primary importance immediately prior to birth.

Her labor will not necessarily be as she imagined it. Her labor will probably not duplicate her visualizations or preparations for sensation.

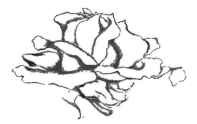

Her responses will not be entirely predictable to her; they will surprise her to the extent that she holds onto set expectations or process and performance of her laboring experience.

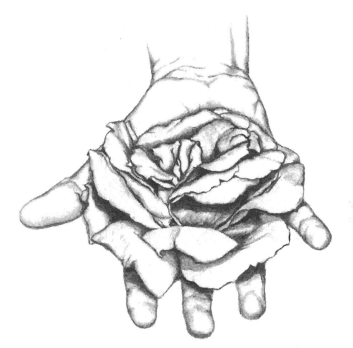

Labor is two people working together, mother and baby. A mother must yield to wherever her baby takes her in labor. Preparation and plans have been of the mother's making. Now she must open herself to the unknown of her baby travelling through her. Her work is hard and requires access to her own strength, and it is easy, because she can only follow her baby. There is no other choice. It is this combination of strength and yielding that brings a woman through birth in a manner in which she is able to learn more about herself. Whatever the delivery experience, whatever the outcome, it is a learning experience of great potential for the woman, one from which she can glean valuable insight into herself, if she is not afraid to look.

The courage to look inside at the unknown country that

stretches beyond our current knowing is the same quality of "letting go", of yielding necessary for birthing ourselves and our babies.

This philosophy has been communicated throughout classes — that a woman is preparing for the unknown, and once she is prepared, she is still before the doorway to the unknown. However, she is calm and relaxed at the entrance. She accepts the unknown and accepts her inability to control it, necessitating her yielding to it. Her strength lies in her confidence to open the door and begin the journey through unknown territory. This confidence influences the journey itself. This is especially true for a woman giving birth for the first time. Working through fears, conflicts, and anxieties has given her the confidence to open the door. It has not given her any more knowledge of what is there for her. Only her labor can tell her more.

Section III
Mind-Body Integration

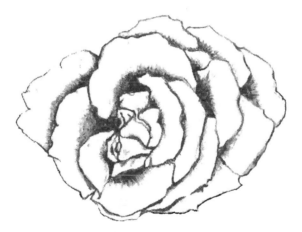

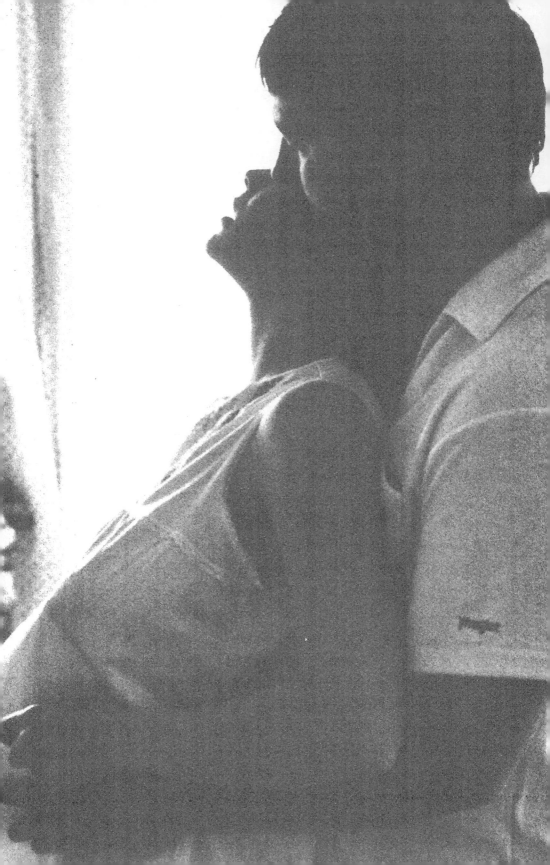

Chapter Nine

Resolving Complications

THE BENEFITS OF psychotherapy in resolving conflict have already been discussed to a limited extent. The practice of long or brief term psychotherapy when indicated definitely contributes towards uncomplicated birth.[1]

Within the context of the actual birth, particular psychological interventions may be employed for augmentation of normal labor and delivery if the practitioner is knowledgeable of her/his field and has an understanding of psychological process and application. The importance of psychological training in order to grasp an awareness of psychological process is necessary, if a practitioner is to avoid the limited conceptual framework of medical training. Training in psychology is necessary in order to apply concepts of responsibility and self-determination to physical process. Well-meaning practitioners with an "alternative bent" to their philosophy of medicine are sometimes the most disrespecting of a client's psychological process. This occurs mostly because of an inability to identify psychological process, thereby falling unwittingly into the role of "Saviour", responsible for curing the illness or problem being presented to them by the client. The rescue triangle[2] becomes a reality, with the practitioner playing the role of rescuer of the client from his/her malady or unpleasant situation. In the case of childbirth, the client gives away her responsibility to the practitioner, along with the power to correct the situation, and waits for the midwife or physician to deliver the desired outcome. The practitioner in such a situation will often end up being the "villain" in the eyes of the client when he/she is unable to deliver the "goods", since in fact it is only the client herself that can give birth.

A study of psychology is necessary for a medically trained

practitioner to identify psychological process, both his/her own and the client's. The practitioner will be unable to apply the psychological interventions discussed in this chapter without the ability to identify beliefs within a client's highly integrated psychological process. The following discussion presumes an ability to understand psychological process in order to identify conflictual beliefs and incongruencies present within an intact and functioning belief system.

Theory of the Double Bind

A double bind is a resulting outcome of paradoxical communication which presents commands or instructions, which in the psychological situation are mutually exclusive and therefore contradictory. In the therapeutic situation the instructions are on the surface contradictory, but in actuality each instruction leads to the same outcome or goal. In the therapeutic situation, the goal has already been defined by the client, who has entered into a relationship with a professional in order to achieve the identified goal. For purposes of this book, the outcome is defined as normal delivery, without medical intervention, or "natural childbirth" as the client identifies it.

The theory of double bind to explain schizophrenia is well documented in psychological literature.[3] It will be beneficial to include a brief discussion of the brain and its functioning, in order to illustrate the hypnotic quality of paradoxical communications. Both the pathological and the therapeutic situations will be described.

Dominant and Non-Dominant Hemisphere Communication

Simply stated, the brain can be divided into 2 hemispheres, the dominant (almost always the left side) and the non-dominant (right) hemispheres. The dominant hemisphere is actively involved in verbal, digital or analytical thinking, while the non-dominant hemisphere processes non-verbal communication such as body language which accounts for feelings, hunches, and intuition.

In a schizophrenogenic family situation, a child may be receiving double messaged communication on a consistent basis. A message such as "I am not angry" is processed on a verbal content level by the dominant hemisphere. Non verbal communication, such as the father slamming his fist down on the table as he says, "I am not angry" is processed simultaneously by the child's non-dominant hemisphere. The child, while indoctrinated in the emphasis of reality placed on the verbal content, cannot easily analyze the communication in order to become aware of the reason for his/her confusion about the message given by the father. The child senses the anger as it is processed by the non-dominant hemisphere (fist slamming down on table, loud voice) and also processes the unspoken signal of danger over disagreement with the father. The dominant hemisphere processes the content of the words, "I am not angry." Confusion is the result.

An ongoing conflict/inner confusion takes place when a 30-year-old woman, Mary, is faced with the following untenable situation during a therapy hour as she attempts to "please" her father:

message no. 1 (15 minutes into the session)
Father: "It touches me that Mary needs me to help her out financially. I feel a kind of closeness with her as a father; that my daughter still needs me."

message no. 2 (20 minutes later)
Father (turning to his wife): "She's 30 years old now. When the hell is she going to be independent and take care of herself?"

In the above situation, Mary is given the instructions, as she has been throughout her childhood, "Be independent" and "Be dependent." There is no way to follow either instruction successfully without failing at the other one. The result is confusion, which in the extreme is a schizophrenic individual attempting to follow both communications simultaneously. In such a situation withdrawal may be the resolution chosen to escape the state of painful confusion. In the less extreme case is the neurotic, alternating contradictory behavior in an attempt to successfully please by carrying out both communications in a cyclic manner.

Only through awareness of the double-messaged communication is the individual able to step outside of the paradoxical framework. By identifying the "crazy" communication a person is free to choose not to respond to either message. It is easy to understand a child's inability to do this in a family situation.

Within the framework of responding to a double bind, by attempting to follow both instructions, the individual is unaware of the 2 messages being communicated. This is also true of the person giving the communication.

For this reason, communication theory has been one of the most effective theories used in the treatment of schizophrenics when application in the form of family therapy is accessible as a mode of treatment. Johnson further illustrates the double bind as leading to schizophrenia in childhood:

> *When children perceive anger and hostility of a parent, as they did on many occasions, immediately the parent would deny the anger and would insist that the child deny it too, so that the child was faced with the dilemma of whether to believe the parent or his own senses. If he believed his senses, he maintained a firm grasp on reality; if he believed the parent, he maintained the needed relationship, but distorted his perception of the reality. (p. 143)[4]*

By distorting reality, the child may also distort or block his perception of all non-dominant hemisphere communication.

The Therapeutic Double Bind

In the therapeutic double bind, a psychotherapist and client have come together for a particular goal for which the client has employed the therapist to help him achieve. Let us examine the example of a man coming in because he is suffering from headaches, which have been determined to have no physical basis. The client assumes no control of his situation; he sees himself a victim of the condition.

During the course of treatment, one objective in therapy will be to let him discover that he does have control over his headaches, as this will be a necessary precursor to eliminating them. Therefore, the therapist gives the following paradoxical instruction: "Before we attempt to deal with the situation about your headaches, it is important to give your body permission to have them, as they may be necessary at this time. This way we will not attempt to move too fast, as this is a delicate situation. Therefore, it will be helpful if during this first week of therapy, you increase your headaches to (x number) per day."

The above intervention is termed "prescribing the symptom." If the client responds by not having more headaches, he is told that he has succeeded in controlling his headaches. He has not "performed the instructions" and is therefore in control. If he responds by having an increased number of headaches, he has also succeeded, in control of his headaches. If he responds in opposition, and has no headaches at all, he has succeeded in alleviating his symptoms, and may then change the goal of his therapy, as he has already succeeded in eliminating his headaches.

In either of the first 2 responses, the client will succeed in the objective intended by the therapist. Without an awareness of the therapist's specific intent, the client remains within the framework of the paradoxical communication and cannot fail at being in control, no matter what his response.

Prescribing a relapse of depression for a client who has succeeded at making her way out of the depressive state is indicated if fear of failure, or actual perceived failure, is determined to be a significant causal factor in the depression itself. By instructing a person in the probability of a relapse as a normal, common occurrence, the fear of failure is alleviated, and a relapse rarely occurs in my experience. Since it is already permissible, the client has nothing to fail at, and is relieved of the anxiety of failure which is in fact a causal factor of the depression. Prescribing a relapse is another form of paradoxical communication.

Use of Double Bind as a Psychotherapeutic Intervention in Labor

In the former examples of therapeutic double bind, objectives and goals were illustrated. Working towards objectives can be a means to the end goal. It is necessary for a practitioner to distinguish goals from objectives in order to stimulate motivation and bypass resistance. By treating a double bind with respect to an objective, the goal was achievable. The goal is defined and agreed upon by both client and practitioner. The objective is defined by the practitioner through professional knowledge and understanding of his/her field. To the client's perception, the said "objective" appears to be a goal.

In the following example, the goal defined is natural childbirth. The objective defined is use of anesthesia or analgesia.

Karen was a 21-year-old woman expecting her first baby, desiring a natural birth in an alternative birth center. Karen was ambivalent about living with the father of the child, and at the time of labor was living at her mother's house, considering the prospect of single motherhood.

Karen had taken classes, seemingly to gain a sense of confidence. However, throughout her pregnancy she remained in a childlike role, very dependent on her health practitioners.

When she began labor, Karen clung to the labor support people (labor coaches) asking for medication to take the pain away. The midwife told Karen that she could be given medication when the contractions got stronger and she was farther along in her labor. As her contractions picked up in intensity and her labor progressed, the midwife told her that when contractions got very strong, her labor would be nearly over. However, meanwhile she was told to make them stronger in order to progress to the point at which she could be medicated. When contractions become "stronger" Karen was told she did not need medication as her labor was almost finished.

Karen gave birth naturally, and was extremely grateful for not having received medication when she had asked for it. Instructions to make contractions harder and more effective in order to obtain medication enabled Karen to continue working through labor rather than falling into panic or despair. She was able to continue in her objective towards medication which resulted in her long planned goal of natural birth.

Each communication, i.e. (1) When contractions are stronger you will get medication and (2) When contractions are strong labor will be nearly over (and there will be no need for medication) are exclusive of the other. However, both were congruent with the activity of increasing the strength of contractions. The midwife used the objective of medication as incentive to make contractions stronger (in order to avoid uterine inertia). As this instruction was followed, labor progressed to the point of delivery, with no medication necessary. The means by which medication would be accessible (by having strong contractions), was defined as the same means by which birth occurs naturally. The goal, as defined by the client upon entering the relationship with the practioner(s) was achieved by the client herself. This is an important point of confidence for the mother and effects her bonding experience with the infant immediately after birth.

A second illustration of a double bind, used to resolve uterine inertia, unfolds in the following case example.

Colleen was a 33-year-old Caucasian woman expecting her 3rd child. Her daughter was 3 years old at the time of delivery and had been her 2nd child. Her first child, born 10 years before her daughter, had been adopted out. Her husband and father of her 3-year-old daughter, expressed ambivalence about being present during the actual birth. Colleen, however, strongly desired his presence at the birth of their second child, as she felt she had missed her husband's presence at the birth of their daughter. Her husband reluctantly attended childbirth classes and stayed with her during the first part of her labor until her contractions began to be ineffective at opening her cervix.

Colleen's contractions began to be ineffective at 4 centimeters, and she remained at 4 centimeters for 4 hours. The husband was sent out, finally, at Colleen's request, which eliminated a source of anxiety—her need not to scare him and to give him a "nice time." She had developed uterine inertia. Colleen proclaimed that the baby was just too big, and that she could not get it out. She demanded a Cesarean setion. The physician attending her told her that he would look into arranging a Cesarean section, but that it would take some time to set up, and that in the meantime it would be beneficial for the contractions to start up again, as contractions stimulate the baby's lungs, making it healthier and ready for breathing when it is born. He explained how this was especially important for babies that are to be born by Cesarean section, as they benefit from the stimulation of hard contractions since they are not massaged through the birth canal, which also prepares a baby's lungs for breathing at birth.

Within 20 minutes Colleen's contractions started up again, strong and firm, and 40 minutes later she delivered a 9 lb. healthy baby boy, with a 2nd phase of less than 5 minutes.

Colleen responded to the instruction to have hard contractions in order to have a healthy baby by Cesarean section. However as her contractions continued, Colleen gave birth vaginally, achieving her initially stated goal of natural healthy delivery.

The objective defined in this example was a healthy baby, which included the presence of strong and continued contractions. Strong contractions were also the means by which she could enable herself to birth vaginally, even though she had thought of herself as too small to deliver the 9 lb. baby boy. The means to the objective are identical to the means to the goal. Colleen was delighted at the outcome of her contractions, and immediately bonded to her son, in the presence of her husband who came in minutes after delivery.

The above example identifies the power of limiting beliefs (i.e., I am too small to birth my baby) as affecting the labor process. By going with her resistance, by agreeing with her, the physician was able to use the power of her resistance itself to birth her baby. Through agreement and informing her of the importance of continued contractions to stimulate the baby's lungs, he was able to stimulate her motivation for a healthy baby. This is the same principle of "going with the resistance" that is used in judo. Rather than stopping the opponent's resistance with direct blockage, a judo expert positions his/her body in such a way as to put the force of the coming blow back onto the opponent, thereby actually using the force of the resistance. This same principle of dealing with resistance is documented in psychotherapeutic literature.[5]

Again in this case, the 2 communications, (1) I am going to look into arranging a C-section (since you are not having contractions) and (2) You can continue to have contractions for the baby's health, were mutually exclusive on the surface. However it bears repeating that the means to the objective (healthy baby after C-section) were identical to the means to the goal of natural childbirth. To achieve either one, strong contractions were necessary. The double bind was a successful intervention. Had it not been, and CPD were diagnosed,* the baby's lungs would have in fact been better prepared for breathing after Cesarean section. Therefore, either way the outcome would have meant success for the woman giving birth.

Manipulation of the Environment for Effective Birthing and the Use of Indirect Hypnosis for Prevention of Hemorrhage

The manipulation of the environment has been mentioned previously as a means of intervention in labor. The following case further illustrates the psychological components of such intervention through the example of a single mother who maintained a sense of strength and belief in herself, but lacked an ability to yield easily to support from others.

Lonnie was a 27-year-old single woman expecting her first child. She was an athlete, training extensively before becoming

---

*CPD is cephalo pelvic disproportion which means that the pelvic bones are considered to be too small to birth the baby through.

pregnant. She continued to lead a very active life throughout her pregnancy, and was extemely healthy and physically strong.

During the middle part of her pregnancy, Lonnie became somewhat upset and confused by her body image. She saw herself as getting big and clumsy, unable to move in the manner in which she was used to moving. During a prenatal interview, she surprised herself by bursting into tears about her changing body image and her feeling that the father of the child was not interested in the baby. She struggled to resolve her feelings about her ex-lover, which she did by rejecting him, deciding she could be strong without him and didn't need him. She then turned her attention to her feelings about her body image, and was gradually able to accept her body and to adjust to various limitations of activities, excelling in other activities including bicycling and hiking. However, there remained present in her belief system, a belief in femininity or yielding as weak and distasteful to some extent. Her belief in womanhood as strong and powerful would be an asset to her in labor. However, her strength in her identity as a feminist did not easily incorporate the experience of pregnancy and birth. This accounted for the conflict evident during the 2nd trimester of pregnancy. Although this incongruency of belief was resolved to a large extent during the 3rd trimester, Lonnie had to work through it again in her labor. (Review of Chapter II, "The Effect of Belief and Attitude on the Labor Process" will be helpful to the reader in understanding Lonnie, especially with respect to the incorporation of pregnancy and birth into the definition of womanhood.)

Lonnie needed the support of friends for a longer period of time than she had thought she would. For Lonnie it was important that she be in close physical proximity to her labor coach (a good female friend) from 2 centimeters on. It became apparent that Lonnie really needed a great deal of support even in early labor, in order to relax and not "push" the process. As a woman of great strength she tended to rely heavily on her strength but found it difficult to yield to relaxation and waiting for labor to progress at her body's own speed. Her impatience and desire to push the baby out with sheer strength of muscle became particularly evident in second stage of labor. It was necessary to involve 4-5 people actively in supporting her physically so that she could soften and yield to her body process. During 2nd stage, Lonnie began pushing so hard with each contraction that her cervix tightened and the baby was being forced backwards into the uterus. Her thighs and calves were tight with the kind of muscular strength that took her cross country on a bike or up a steep mountain in the

Sierras. It was during 2nd stage that Lonnie had to learn the yielding and softness of her femininity which she had until this time largely negated as "weak," and lost behind the advocation of the strength and power of womanhood. What Lonnie needed to incorporate into her beliefs of strength in womanhood was the ability to accept support from others in order to let go in birth.

In between and during contractions Lonnie was encouraged to let her body go totally limp and to not push. Between contractions she would crouch in a knee chest position with people supporting any muscle that needed to be held in order for her to totally release control of it. During a contraction, Lonnie was physically supported by 2 people, one on each side and under either arm, bracing her as she pitched her body forward from a kneeling position with knees spread wide apart. Lonnie needed to let others completely support her body in order to relax enough to yield to the baby coming down her vagina.

With a woman who experienced the opposite problem, of becoming too dependent on others, unable to activate her own strength, the above environmental intervention would not have been conducive to labor. It is necessary to understand the psychological process of the client, in order to manipulate the environment to the woman's advantage for getting access to the particular resource needed. Assessing what is lacking is of utmost importance, and being able to recognize the needed resource will then dictate the intervention required.

After Lonnie had relinquished her body to others for support, in order to relax during the period of not pushing, her baby had begun to come down again into the vagina. At this point we were able to help Lonnie retain her ability to relax and let go, while she gradually began pushing during contractions, only with her uterus and diaphragm, letting everything else remain loose.

At this point Lonnie was making steady progress in pushing her baby down, as she had learned to push effectively, rather than against herself. She was no longer pushing with sheer muscle strength, attempting to birth her baby instantaneously as she had been doing earlier. She was yielding to the time that her body would take, in order to give birth. During the process of learning that took place Lonnie had expended great energy and was visibly fatigued. It is possible that the fatigue itself was conducive to her yielding. As I watched Lonnie continue in her labor, I felt the occurrence of hemorrhage as a strong possibility considering the incongruencies of belief that had to be worked through, the physical effort that had been expended in doing so, and the general "working through" of incorporation of pregnancy and birth into her identity as a woman.

It was important that I did not speak or direct Lonnie in any way towards being strong or gaining access to her strength at that time, as it would not be conducive to the yielding process that was now underway. However I felt it imperative in preventing a hemorrhage at home to begin laying the foundations for her gaining access to her resource of strength immediately after birth. I therefore whispered into her ear with emphasis on particular words for increased hypnotic effect, the assertion that she would have a surge of great strength and energy at the time her baby would be born. I told her that this was always true and simply a natural phenomenon. I repeated this several times throughout the duration of the labor, sometimes during a contraction and sometimes in between.

As Lonnie gave birth to a 7 lb. baby girl, there was a spurt of blood which covered much of the baby's body, and the placenta followed soon after, with continued bleeding. I immediately told Lonnie that her uterus would clamp down very hard and fast when she held her baby. I placed emphasis through tone of voice on particular words, again for hypnotic effectiveness, and used the hypnotic technique of coupling one event (holding the baby) to a particular activity (uterus clamping down), maximizing the autonomic response through communication to the non-dominant hemisphere.[6]

Lonnie's bleeding decreased to a trickle as she took her baby, and I continued to repeat the instruction of clamping down the uterus. Bleeding stopped soon after, except for normal discharge.

Lonnie indeed perked up right as her baby was born and exclaimed at how good and strong she felt. She told me one month later, that she remembered me telling her about the surge of energy she would get when her baby was born, and that during labor she found it hard to believe yet clung to the idea because it made her feel good, and was very happy when she found it to be true for her.

Lonnie did not remember me giving her instructions to clamp down her uterus. She did remember, however, an image from a movie she had seen in which the doctor had insisted a woman stop bleeding after birth because she lived high on a mountain, and he was unable to get her to any medical facility. Lonnie said that she had a very clear image of this scene in her head, with the woman stopping her bleeding.

The fact that Lonnie did not remember my instructions, but remembered the scene from the movie which carried the same message, is evidence of the hypnotic effect of my instructions. The message was communicated directly to the non-dominant hemisphere (subconscious), surfacing in consciousness with the scene from the movie. The subconscious is associated with the automatic processes of the body, or the autonomic nervous system which includes contractions of the uterus, breathing, the beating of the heart, etc. Contractions of the uterus are stimulated by oxytocin which is released from the anterior pituitary gland in the limbic system.

The limbic system in this manner acts as a relay between emotions and physical process, as emotions may be registered physically by release, inhibition, or alteration in hormonal output. The hormone oxytocin in general increases in amount being made in the pituitary in the presence of anger, and decreases in the presence of fear.

The above case history illustrates the need for the ability to assess the mind-body relationship in any given moment, always remembering that in the present lies the power of change or potentiality in any direction. The direction that labor takes can offer increased ability to ascertain potential for complications, as it did in Lonnie's case. Observing her process as it became actualized in labor rendered immediate information about the potential for postpartun hemorrhage. Laying foundations for increased energy after birth increased the probability of the instruction to "clamp down the uterus" to be effective when given postpartum. In this manner, her strength could be activated as a resource at the correct time, without interfering with the 2nd stage of labor when she needed to yield to the baby coming down through her vagina.

Hypnotic suggestion is a necessary tool for the practitioner using a psychophysiological approach. Full comprehension of this art is beyond the scope of this book. It is sufficient to point out that hypnotic suggestion may also be called non-dominant hemisphere communication, which we all engage in. We are always communicating to both the dominant (through verbal content) and non-dominant (through tonality, pattern of speech, etc.) hemispheres simultaneously, sometimes congruently and sometimes incongruently. Indirect hypnosis is simply the art of consciously communicating and being aware of what is being communicated to the non-dominant hemisphere. The practitioner's use of indirect hypnosis also presumes a goal which has been agreed upon by the practitioner and client at the time they enter into a contractual agreement in order to meet that goal. The art of indirect hypnosis is the ability to facilitate a given person's resources for meeting his/her goal. Further study of this art is necessary for the serious practitioner desiring greater effectiveness through a psychophysiological approach. The literature on neurolinguistic programming[7] is a good beginning, but should be embarked on only after a basic study of psychological process has been completed.

Summary of Environmental Interventions

Alterations of environment to affect psychophysiological process include:

(1) Clearing the room of people, withdrawing support, in order to have access to an individual's strength (as in the case of Heather in Chapter II.)

(2) Increasing the amount of physical support in order to bring out the opposite resource of yielding (as with Lonnie).

(3) Creating absolute quiet in between contractions to facilitate deep relaxation and absorption into the labor process.

(4) Creating distraction in between contractions to facilitate the body process of labor may be effective for the neurotic. Such distraction may serve to circumvent the paralysis that can accompany severe approach-avoidance conflict, common in neurosis.

(5) Use of the toilet. As mentioned in an earlier case history,* the bathroom is a place in which most of us have repeatedly experienced letting go of the sphincter muscles in the urethra and anus. Because of this physical association, which may perhaps even constitute a conditioned reflex, it can be advantageous for a woman to sit on the toilet during contractions. When used as an intervention, sitting on the toilet has increased the strength and hardness of contractions for some women. If the woman is sexually inhibited during labor, or romantically inclined, and experiencing uterine inertia, the environment of the bathroom and the act of sitting on the toilet may break the romantic atmosphere, precipitating hard contractions. Sitting on the toilet, particularly if labor is stopped at 7-10 cms. or in second stage, may increase pressure on the rectum, bladder, and vagina, which further reinforces the conditioned response to let go of the sphincter muscles themselves. The desire to push may also be

---

*See Chapter V.

enhanced, and effectiveness of pushing may greatly increase on the toilet when no other position has yielded any progress.

(6) Performing "parent-ectomies" or other "relative-" or "friend-ectomies" when appropriate: There may be present at the birth a particular person(s) who puts the woman into conflict or performance anxiety which can affect the labor. When this occurs, removal of that particular person may resolve uterine inertia. This is particularly true for performance anxiety which elicits a fear response of some degree. Fear has the potential of significantly decreasing oxytocin, thus increasing possibility of uterine intertia. It may also be necessary when there is severe marital discord. (This might be called a "spouse-ectomy"). Parents are usually the most common offenders. Performance anxiety in general seems to be highest when a parent is present. However, this is only a generalization, and is also culturally affected. For example, in the black culture, a mother's presence is often very positive and supportive, as is true in the Chicano culture, to a large extent. However, as each of these cultures lose their individual identities and merge with the white, middle-class, American culture, there are greater deviations from the initial norm. Individual assessment is always necessary for each woman. In recognition of individuality lies the strength and accuracy of the psychophysiological assessment process as described in this book.

The Phenomenological Approach

In view of the interventions described in this chapter, it is necessary to remain conscious of the uniqueness of each and every woman for which these interventions might take place. It is necessary to study the belief system of each woman, in order to assess what effect any intervention might have for her. An understanding of a particular woman's beliefs and the relationship between her beliefs and her family system can be best achieved through a phenomenological approach whereby description of the woman takes place without prior assumptions or interpretations of what her actions, words, or behavior might mean. Rather her manner of being in the world is described as completely individual to her. For example, chronic vaginitis may express for one woman mostly rage towards her husband, while for another the same physical manifestation may express an irritation with motherhood (or anything else that the woman associates with irritation in her vagina). Uterine inertia in one woman may be an expression of something totally different than in another, as we have seen throughout this book. Prenatal classes address our culture's beliefs.

Psychological process as presented in this book is simply a manner of being in the world which can be described from simple observation. This brings us back to the basic premise of this book; that a woman gives birth as she lives. Being able to describe and identify this manner of being-in-the-world may enable us to intervene in such a way as to increase the choices available to a particular woman. Patterns of being-in-the-world are not totally predictable, as the potential of creativity in the present always exists. New choices for adjusting to labor and birth are always available within an expansion of that same style or manner of living described. However, the greater our knowledge of the manner of being-in-the-world for an individual, and the more accurate our description of these patterns of being-in-the-world has on the woman as she relates to her body process, the more therapeutic can the practitioner be in intervening. Intervention is aimed at expanding a woman's accessibility to her resources. Through psychotherapy, a woman may increase her resources, as is true in classes. However, during the labor process itself, interventions are aimed more at making resources which may be hidden from the woman, accessible, and not increasing resources. This does not mean that an increase in resources could not take place in labor, it is only less probable, though the potential still exists.

Given that attention to the uniqueness of the individual is of utmost importance, the clinical judgment for the appropriate intervention has unique application to the particular woman. Interventions discussed in this chapter are meant to be applied within this phenomenological philosophy.[8] The effect of an intervention needs to be weighed with respect to the effect on the labor process for an individual woman. Existential phenomenology as applied to medicine simply enables the practitioner a framework large enough to encompass each individual without prior assumption or theory which would limit the actual perception of that person's reality. The categories of beliefs affecting labor (Chapter II) are artificial divisions which exist for teaching purposes, but are to be applied with flexibility to individual women.

Consistent with the phenomenological approach is the description of case examples. Within these individual examples is present the clarity of belief systems and relationship of belief to mind and body which become physically expressed.

REFERENCES

1. Mehl, L. and Peterson, G. An Existential Approach to Prenatal Risk Screening. In Ahmed, P. (ed) *Psychosocial Aspects of Pregnancy*. New York: Elsevier-North Holland, 1981.

2. For further information on the psychodynamics created in a rescue situation see: Steiner, C. The Rescue Triangle. *Issues in Radical Therapy*, Vol. 1 no. 4, Fall 1973.

3. Watzlawick, P. *Change*. New York, W. W. Norton Co., 1974.

4. Johnson, A. et al. Studies of Schizophrenia at the Mayo Clinic. 11. Observations on Ego Functions in Schizophrenia. *Psychiatry*, 19:143-148, 1956.

5. Hayley, J. *Problem Solving Therapy*. San Francisco, Jossey-Bass Publishers, 1977.

6. Grinder, J. Bandler, R. and DeLozier, J. *Patterns of the Hypnotic Technique of Milton H. Erickson, M.D.* Vols. I and II, Cupertino, Meta Publications, 1977.

7. Bandler, R. and Grinder J. *The Structure of Magic*, Vols. I and II. Palo Alto, Science and Behavior Books, 1976.

8. Boss, M. *Existential Foundations of Medicine and Psychology*. New York, Aronson, 1979.

Chapter Ten

Psychosexual Changes

A HEALTHY PREGNANCY includes a healthy psychosexual development. A healthy pregnancy is one in which a woman is free
to enjoy her body, to experience the sensuality and sexuality of
another being growing within her. As healthy psychosexual
development is rare in our culture, so is pregnancy free of some
conflict about sexuality a relative rarity.

Pregnancy is a period of radical change, and may be
accompanied by changes in life style. It is a time of stress which
magnifies the problem areas in our lives. As such, it is a
tremendous opportunity for psychological growth and
integration. Sexuality is an area which rarely escapes conflict at
some level, since sex education for the young, and
acknowledgement of sexuality as a part of healthy functioning is
relatively new to middle class America. Beliefs in sex as "dirty" or
"bad" which have been learned in early childhood, may intensify
or re-surface as a woman feels her body moving towards
motherhood. For the male partner as well, sex with his female
partner may be different to him now that she is becoming a
mother. Dichotomies between motherhood and sexuality are not
unusual, and can take their toll on the relationship between the
woman and man. Free and enjoyable access to one another's bodies
may become forbidden, as motherhood looms on the horizon.
Interpretations of motherhood have not always included
sexuality.

The Bible itself has been misinterpreted by various religions as
condemning sexuality rather than condemning adultery.*

*Sex within the realm of marital relationship is to be enjoyed according to Proverbs 5: 18-19,
while adultery is seen to degrade the experience according to Romans 1:25-27.

Description of sex as degrading within the context of extramarital relations for many worshippers became the emotional belief in sex itself as degrading and dirty. This is the same association which has been taught throughout our present day culture.

Progesterone increases during pregnancy accentuate both oral and sexual conflict. Oral conflicts, when present, are revived. Ordinary nausea may become extreme. Eating food, taking nourishment into the fetus may become conflictual if the pregnant woman experiences difficulties in identifying as a mother, or if her childhood experience of being mothered was negative. Hostility towards a woman's own mother may predispose her to increased difficulty in eating during early pregnancy, beyond the normal 1st trimester nausea. Such conflict may increase stress to a point where spontaneous abortion is the result. For such women, vomiting is often felt to be a means of getting rid of the baby on a subliminal level. An 80% success rate has been achieved in maintaining pregnancies for women who are identified as habitual aborters, when the issue of conflict in motherhood is dealt with in psychotherapy.[1]

Pregnancy reawakens a woman's own experience of being mothered. Her perceptions of her own mother as a positive or negative figure in her life are particularly influential in the first time mother, who has not been presented with a previous opportunity for integration of motherhood into her identity. The woman's perception of her father's response to her mother's pregnancies and to motherhood in general, is also an important learning experience in childhood. Whether her father's responses towards motherhood were perceived as positive or negative by her, will influence her ability to integrate motherhood into her identity within a framework of male-female relationship. Learned attitudes towards womanhood in general will also influence this integration.

Fear of losing a husband through pregnancy may also present conflict, especially if this association has proven true in the woman's original family, or if she perceives it in her husband's family history.

Pregnancy makes the sexual act visible and sexual conflicts already present are magnified. The rise in estrogen in pregnancy generally increases sexual drive in women, therefore bringing them face to face with existing sexual conflict as this drive increases.

Artificial divisions have existed between sexuality, childbirth, and other life events. Both sex and birth have been kept divided from the rest of life. Mystery, myths, and false formulations have arisen to explain both, in the absence of acceptance of these areas of human experience as normal, healthy activities.

The cultural purpose of the clinical atmosphere and traditional procedures during labor and birth in this country can be viewed as that of maintaining the artificial division between sexuality and birth. Shaving pubic hair, sterile drapes, and routine episiotomies all serve to hide from a woman and the hospital staff the fact that birth is sexual. It is no wonder that as we have culturally alienated a woman from her genitals, that this alienation would continue to be perpetrated in a social institution such as a hospital. It also makes obvious the difficulty that can arise as women experience the vulnerability of exposing the vagina and genital area of the body during birth.

There is some evidence to suggest that labor and birth may need to be painful in order for a woman in our sexually inhibited culture to lose her sexual inhibitions for birth. Warren Gadpaille, in his book *Cycles of Sex,* cites evidence that in cultures in which sexuality is accepted as a part of life as early as childhood, childbirth is experienced as easier and *less* painful. (This does not necessarily mean "no pain.")

From this evidence, one could hypothesize that in sexually repressed cultures, a prolonged and painful labor may be symptomatic of the fight against the sexuality of the experience. The greater the fight, the greater the increase in stress. Likewise, the more stress experienced around the conflict of sexuality, during birth, the greater the occurrence of complication due to the accumulation of stress. Accumulation of stress could express itself in a number of different ways, including fetal distress, maternal high blood pressure, uterine inertia, or hemorrhage. Stress is a very real physicalization of psychological disparity.

Gadpaille further cites evidence of an easier adjustment to breastfeeding, the more accepting the culture is of the normal sexual components of motherhood. In such cultures it is natural for the mother to enjoy the sexual stimulation of her infant's suckling, and to stimulate the genitalia of her infant for the infant's pleasure as she changes a diaper. For the infant's normal development, it is important that the mother's acts be fairly consistent with the norms of the culture, otherwise conflict could result as the infant became socialized in childhood.

In early classes and throughout pregnancy, an education to sexuality as a part of birth and mothering and as a healthy body process is important. Specifically, information regarding the hormone oxytocin can be particularly enlightening for both women and men. Oxytocin is the hormone released during labor, during sexual orgasm, and during the "let down" reflex in breastfeeding.* This information alone can sometimes give a woman the right to her sexuality through her body hormones. Guilt may have left her unable to recognize feelings of sensuality associated with birth or breastfeeding. Through knowledge about this similarity between labor, breastfeeding, and orgasm a woman may feel free of former guilt. Mothers can indeed be sexual, enjoying their bodies in motherhood as a form of healthy sexuality.

The following case history further illustrates the interference of conflict in sexuality as it relates to motherhood and breastfeeding.

Sonja was a 24 year old Christian, who had given birth to twin boys by Cesarean section. One month after birth her milk supply began decreasing to the point at which she needed to begin supplemental formula feedings in order for her babies to gain the normal amount of weight. They had begun to lose weight by the end of one month.

Sonja came in for a relaxation visualization with the goal of increasing her milk supply. She very much wanted to feed her twins solely on breast milk and felt that if she could relax, she might be able to produce more milk for her babies.

Sonja was able to relax easily, and when the relaxation induction was complete, found herself able to visualize her breasts. She described her breasts as soft and round, tender and warm. It became evident in the course of her description, that her concept of motherhood did not include the sensuality of the breastfeeding experience that her two sons elicited on a biological level. Because of a strong Christian belief system which in her experience divided sexuality from motherhood, Sonja found herself in conflict between her bodily sensations elicited by the nursing process, and her image of a good Christian mother. The fact that her twins were boys increased this anxiety, resulting in an inhibition in the hormone oxytocin, in order to resolve the conflicting images of sexuality and motherhood.

Using Sonja's belief system, I explained to her the significances of God's design of her body. I told her that the fact of oxytocin

---

*The "let down" reflex is the biological reflex which releases milk from the breast to the baby.

being the identical hormone that is released during lovemaking as is released in breastfeeding was certainly no accident on God's part, and to trust that the similarity in sensation is natural, and meant to be. This type of re-education on an emotional level was important in relieving Sonja of the guilt she experienced around her bodily sensation of breastfeeding. As she re-learned the naturalness of her body's process, Sonja explained that now she could understand why she was drenched in milk during lovemaking, which had previously puzzled her. She had wondered why she could have a "let-down" reflex and an abundance of milk at that time, and yet experience difficulty with her "let-down" reflex when feeding her twins.

During the visualization, it was apparent that Sonja would need further work in order to re-learn her image of motherhood to include sexuality/sensuality. The bridging of these two artifically divided images would require further liberation, on Sonja's and her husband's part with regards to their inhibitions about sexuality in general. However further therapy was interrupted as they were moving out of the country within the following two weeks. Follow-through on this case was therefore unavailable; however, success as to the potential for the resolution of this conflict of mind and body in the realm of sexuality was evident. During the visualization session, Sonja's let-down reflex was activated as she imagined herself as a sexual/sensual mothering woman nursing her twins. With encouragement for making these body sensations permissable, Sonja drenched her bra and blouse with milk during the course of the 60 minute therapy hour.

Hormonal changes in pregnancy may also predispose a woman already under stress to vaginal infection. In prolonged vaginitis, unresponsive to medications and douches, there may exist a psychophysiological interplay exacerbating the irritation. Stress with reference to psychological guilt or ambivalence towards sex may be magnified in pregnancy.

Some effects of emotional/psychological stress in pregnancy have been mentioned with reference to women who repeatedly miscarry. Other stress-inducing conflicts in self-image may predispose some women to this physical response. The basic issue of self-worth may be important to assess even outside of the image of motherhood. A woman may experience herself as not worthy enough to actually make and produce a baby through her own body process. A lack of belief in her own basic adequacy may predispose her to not taking care of herself physically, or increase anxiety about her physical conditon. Fears of responsibility, feelings of incompetence, or a serious inner conflict about commitment to motherhood, can all influence a woman's predisposition toward miscarriage. This does not mean that every woman who experiences such a conflict miscarries, as she may have other beliefs for pregnancy which could counter such conflictual beliefs. Nor does every woman who experiences a miscarriage do so for the above reasons. However, a woman who miscarries repeatedly, and wants to maintain a pregnancy,may benefit from attention to the psychological process in achieving her goal.

The onset of premature labor due to environmental stress has been documented with respect to war, and other highly stressful situations. Premature labor may also be due to the presence of a psycho-emotional conflict which has mounted in intensity with the progression of the pregnancy. In such cases, the conflict was often one which the woman was able to ignore during the earlier part of her pregnancy, and was thus left unresolved. As the time of birth draws near, reality is recognized, sometimes in a form of panic, as previously suppressed anxiety surfaces and spirals in the seemingly untenable position the woman then experiences herself in. I have witnessed a form of this kind of panic in a 20 year old woman who denied the reality of her pregnancy during her first trimester, and continued to live her life as if the question of what to do with the baby once it was born (whether to adopt out or keep it) was yet a long way off, with no need to resolve the issue, until at 7 months of pregnancy she suddenly became aware of the closeness of the baby's birth. It was at this point that she became distraught and panic-stricken about her future and the reality of her need to make a decision for or against motherhood at that time of her life. In distress, she finally decided to adopt the baby out, and soon afterwards went into premature labor.

High levels of stress, whether environmental, psychological, or physical, do have an effect on body process. In the view of the philosophy of this book, the relationship between mind, body, and environment is an interconnected one in which each is perceived as affecting the others. The ability to cope with stress of any kind is an important variable for outcome. Through childbirth classes as presented in this book, women are supported in deepening their ability to handle stress by transforming it into a learning or personal growth experience. It is this model for personal growth that can relieve us of a blame or guilt response to the psychophysiological approach. The ability to look within, to take responsibility for what is there, and to love ourselves brings us in touch with the power present in each of us for change and self-fulfillment.

Siblings

The presence of other children in the family, particularly if the woman is expecting her second child and the first child is under 2 years, can present a multiplicity of problems. Some mothers need to be reminded of the fetus *in utero*, in order to take care of themselves sufficiently. A pregnant mother of a small child or baby is still experiencing the needs and wants of her first child. Her bond to her first baby continues to grow, as the maternal hormones flow. Too often, a mother leaves herself little time to enjoy a second (or subsequent) pregnancy, and unwittingly increases the dependency of her first child on her as she reaches term. The ordinary depression and anxiety of the first child is increased when the baby is born, if the mother has not already begun to make space for the second child, by simply taking time for herself.

In some instances, body changes in pregnancy can be traumatic for the pregnant mother, if she is not making room for the second baby and remains dependent on her first baby for validation of her motherhood. The following example illustrates this symbiosis and the problem it poses for the child-to-be.

Anna was a 28 year old woman, pregnant with her second child. During the course of her second pregnancy, Anna was forced to stop nursing her 8 month old daughter. As her pregnancy progressed, her body produced less and less milk. This posed a problem for Anna, as she felt she was "cheating" her first child by not nursing it to the length of time she had previously decided, one to two years. She began to feel animosity towards the fetus for getting in the way of her mothering relationship with her first child. Although Anna professed to want the pregnancy, she found herself in significant psychic upheaval, as she felt her identity of motherhood to her first child threatened.

During her labor, Anna was unable to put her attention on the new baby coming out, and continued to absorb herself in her first child. Her labor did not progress until the child was taken out of the labor room by Anna's husband. Anna was then able to give birth, and responded readily to the baby once it was born. She was able to bond to her new baby and became very engrossed in the process of meeting her new baby. Anna no longer experienced trauma for herself as a mother. However, her first child had great difficulty with adjustment to the new sibling, as she had experienced no preparation for the sudden change in her mother's attentiveness. The trauma had not resolved itself, but had simply been transferred from mother to daughter.

The above case, although presenting greater pathology than is normal for the average woman, serves to exemplify the integration of mothering of a subsequent child as being potentially complicated by the demands of a first child. Again, the woman benefits from becoming aware of her biological mothering of the new baby on the inside, and her right to enjoy each pregnancy as unique. Providing herself with time alone for herself and the fetus can alleviate the potential for feeling split in her loyalties as a mother. In this manner, she is already defining space in the family and in her mothering for the presence of a new baby. With adequate preparation, complication of labor may be avoided by resolving sibling rivalry to some extent in the prenatal course.

The Experience of the Father in Pregnancy

The psychodynamic process of the father-to-be will be discussed as it relates to the couples' dynamics. A detailed description and analysis of the father's experience would be highly interesting, but is beyond the scope of this book.

Feelings of envy, guilt, or alienation may be present for a father-to-be if there is psychic conflict predisposing him to such feelings. Envy of the pregnancy and birth process, or of the fetus itself, is not uncommon. The extent to which the envy becomes a problem in the relationship mirrors the amount of competition present, either between the couple, or between the father and child-to-be.

If a woman is unhappy with the process of pregnancy and birth, the man may experience guilt feelings, which may hamper his ability to relate freely and openly to both the woman and their baby.

One of the most common conflicts for fathers surrounding the birth of the first child, is the fear of losing the woman's love and attention to the baby. This fear is usually symbolic of a very real loss which will take place for the man, as the woman moves into motherhood. In its most exaggerated form, the couple appear to relate to one another in a mother-son relationship. The woman, in need of acting out her fantasy of mothering, has found a man who responds very positively to such nurturing which is sometimes very one sided. As pregnancy progresses, the woman begins to pay more attention to the coming fetus and may expect the man to begin taking care of her in many of the same ways she had previously "mothered" him. Strain becomes evident during the last couple of months of pregnancy, and it is not uncommon for some physical ailment, which has not shown up in years, to recur in the man. Such physical ailments may begin in the third trimester and last through the postpartum course, until the family has made its adjustments, with each member taking on a new role in the system. Commonly, in such cases, the male partner gradually becomes sicklier throughout the woman's pregnancy, becoming quite sickly when the woman is near term. Competition for "mothering" at this time becomes very intense. The following case history illustrates this process.

Kevin and Marla had been married for 6 years when they decided to have a baby. They had been social workers together in the slums of Detroit and had lived through the trauma of neighborhood racial conflict together. They became therapists only 2 years before the birth of their first child. Again, it was a team endeavor. They often spoke of the necessity for one of them to be strong while the other remained weak, and had acquired insight into how they switched these roles with one another throughout their relationship.

As Marla entered her second trimester of pregnancy, she began to lessen the amount of work she was doing with Kevin in their practice. Kevin became anxious about her withdrawal from work, as it brought up his fear of competition for both work in the outside world to support his family, and competition with the growing fetus for Marla's attention and time.

Kevin had begun dieting when Marla first became pregnant. His "dieting" had snowballed as he continued to lose 50 lbs., the same amount of weight as Marla had gained in her pregnancy. Marla was the picture of health and strength as she entered her third trimester, while Kevin was fading fast, with a recurrence of ulcerative colitis. He had not had ulcerative colitis since his first move away from home to college, 13 years earlier.

Kevin appeared increasingly anxious and extremely irritable as his wife grew more pregnant. He became emaciated, unable to gain weight as his ulcerative colitis worsened. As was customary within the birth program they were enrolled in, Kevin and Marla were planning a "birth dinner." The purpose of the "birth dinner" was for everyone planning to be present at the birth to be together, and to learn more about Marla's feelings about their presence at the birth, and what they might do to help at that time.

Marla had arranged for the dinner to take place on a Sunday, 3 weeks prior to her due date. As two of us pulled up to the house for dinner, Marla came running out of the house crying, in a state of fright, saying that Kevin had just "fainted or something." When we entered the house, Kevin was conscious and upright. He said that he thought maybe he had had a seizure. Kevin asked the physician present to describe what a seizure was like. It became evident that Kevin had not had an actual seizure, but had simply fainted because of a dizziness which was not yet explainable. Details of description of grand mal seizure were explained at Kevin's insistance. Kevin had never in his life had a seizure, and from the description given by Marla, it sounded like a fainting spell.

However, in the next 15 minutes, as conversation had begun to return to the topic of the birth dinner, Kevin began slowly turning his head sideways to the right, his eyes rolling upwards to the ceiling, making a gagging sound. He then proceeded to have his first grand mal seizure. An ambulance was called and Kevin was taken to the emergency room of a nearby hospital.

He continued to have seizures until medicated. He remained in the hospital for 2 weeks, developing severe joint swelling and pain. Extensive medical tests uncovered no physical cause for either the joint swelling or the seizures.

Kevin came home 2 weeks before Marla's labor began. Marla proceeded to have a long drawn out labor, as she had believed she would have no pain in labor, and began counting her labor time from her very first contraction. After a 52 hour labor, and a narrow escape from a Cesarean section, Marla gave birth to a 7 lb. baby girl. During her labor, it was necessary to confront Marla to tell her to stop blaming Kevin for the pain, and to simply accept and use the pain to make progress in labor.

One week after the birth Kevin was again hospitalized for severe joint swelling and pain, again of unknown cause. He did not respond to anti-inflammatory agents and at one point in his "postpartum" illness was in critical conditon. Kevin did improve, and was able to return home 3 weeks later.

Unlike his first hospitalization in which Marla had all but lived in his hospital room, during his second hospitalization Marla remained home with the baby, visiting for much shorter periods of time. Both parents remained home during the year that followed the birth; Marla to care for the baby, and Kevin to make a gradual recovery.

The previous example is an extreme one, showing the physical manifestations of raging conflict over fatherhood for one man. The experience of jealousy, abandonment, and fear of competition all played important parts. These feelings, left unrecognized and unexplored, were part of the confusion and chaos which fatherhood stimulated. Kevin's original mother-son relationship and father-son relationship no doubt also played important roles in his inner conflict. As his own journey towards fatherhood brought these hidden conflicts to the surface, Kevin found himself in an intra-psychic battle, unable to define a place for himself as father in his family. The changing relationship with his wife was the crux of his illness. Unable to remain in the "son" position with her, he struggled to become "strong" perhaps even "fatherly." However, within their family system the see-saw effect was in existence. If one were weak, the other could be strong. Marla, however, was not willing to become the weak one. Her image of pregnancy and motherhood was one of health and strength. Kevin's dependency was also being challenged. As he saw Marla's mothering wane throughout the course of the pregnancy, his anxiety grew and expressed itself in physical form.

In milder cases, recurrent asthma in the father-to-be has been observed as the pregnancy progresses. A spontaneous resolution can sometimes occur in the family system which will help to re-define roles and identities as relationships evolve. The absence of the man, on a business or pleasure trip the month before delivery, is often to the mutual benefit of the pregnant woman and father-to-be. Physical distance may give them each the opportunity to re-define themselves, and then to come back together for birth. For the man, it gives him a chance to let go of the desire for "mothering" and puts him in a place of independence and self-sufficiency before the baby enters the family. Fathers, like mothers, also experience surfacing of conflict during pregnancy which can present opportunity for growth.

Sex in Pregnancy

As sex has been the forbidden fruit in our society for some time, it is to be expected that pregnancy and birth will magnify the conflicts and contradictions that are present in the culture. Emotional conflict in the form of guilt, jealousy, or ambivalence may play a significant role in psychosexual responses during pregnancy. In particular, conflict between sexuality and the developing mother role, may inhibit sexual responsiveness for the man as well as the woman. In such cases, heightened eroticism which is evident with the biological increase in estrogen (hormone) during pregnancy, may be upsetting or even frightening to the woman. As her body becomes increasingly sensitive to sexual arousal via hormonal changes, conflict between the mental image of motherhood and the body's desires can produce agitation and difficulty in communication between the partners.

The encouragement for open communication about sexuality in early pregnancy classes can greatly ease the adjustments that may need to occur later in the pregnancy. Changes in positions for sex as the woman becomes larger can be discussed. The therapeutic effect of sharing feelings about sexuality in a group setting presents a role model for couples to continue with at home. Couples counselling can be suggested if further work seems desirable.

Women need encouragement in loving their bodies as they change throughout the 9 month period. Some women may feel unattractive or even ugly, and often a visualization of the process that is taking place within is a necessary precursor to appreciating the beauty of their bodies and their sexuality in pregnancy. Sexual desire is a valuable form of expression during pregnancy. A woman is as alive, as sensual, as sexual as always during this time, and perhaps even more so. As with any other psychic conflict present, however, magnification of psychosexual conflict will occur during pregnancy.

Children at Birth and Sex Education

Sex education begins at birth. This is literally true for children present at the births of their siblings.

In one survey (Peterson and Mehl, 1976) on the sex education of 3-year-olds in a day care setting, children were asked how babies are born.[2] The most common answers were 1) oral regurgitation 2) anal birth 3) the doctor cuts it out. In the survey, children responded to the question of where babies come from with definite ideas, assumptions, and descriptions. It was not a question to which most children felt they did not have an answer. Sadly, the descriptions offered, often in great detail, were usually inaccurate, frightening to the children themselves (as well as to any adult), and demonstrated a distorted view of body-process. At this age, children are particularly interested in how their body works, and are developing mastery of bodily process. The significance at this point in development of viewing birth as a normal, healthy process may be critical. By this time, children have become aware of the biological differences in the sexes and ask many questions about body processes. The physical form of a pregnant woman brings up the normal questioning response from the 2 or 3 year old.

Fears and mystifications present at this age may be simply transferred to the concept of birth, when it is learned that normal delivery means the baby comes out through the vagina. The fears and mystification remain, long after the facts have been discovered. These same emotionally learned fears, present mostly due to the mystification process, become associated with birth and can be felt in the tension and fear surrounding the birth process in many adult women today.

As early as the age of 3 years children have identified the silence that shrouds the subject of sexuality and birth as fearful, alien, unnatural, distasteful. All of these notions are emotionally learned, and must be re-learned in the future, if birth is to be an enjoyable and healthy process.

The children who answered the question about how babies are born accurately, tended towards matter-of-fact presentation, sometimes based on the child's actual experience at the birth of a sibling. The ability of the 2-3 year old to grasp the normalcy of the birth experience is evident.

Given that a family's attitude towards birth and sexuality is one of matter-of-fact normalcy, acceptance of sex and birth is automatic to the child attending the birth. Obviously, if a family holds an attitude towards birth as an abnormal and frightening event, and had their 3 year old at the birth, the result would no doubt be traumatic, as the child's experience would be processed through the attitudes and beliefs of those around him/her. Children learn to a great extent from the attitudes of family members. The sound of yelling during contractions will usually be accepted without apprehension as normal, if it is accepted as so by the father and others attending the birth.

Other factors that create a healthy learning atmosphere for the child have included a) the presence of an adult who is emotionally close to the child and with whom the child feels comfortable and trusting to be the responsible "babysitter" during the birth. This adult's primary focus is the child, and she/he is present to answer any questions or concerns that the child has during the labor and birth process, b) an open door policy that allows the child to be free to come or go presents an opportunity for children to determine their own "readiness" at any particular moment. The support of the adult responsible for the child is again important. Playing with the child outside, or taking him/her out for lunch may be exactly what is appropriate. The child determines the amount of time spent at the labor or birth (given that the mother agrees to the child's presence), and c) appropriate education/preparation prenatally. Talking about the baby *in utero* and illustrating growth of fetus through books, progressing to the event of birth, engages a child's attention and readies him/her for the process.

Children are sexual human beings. Sexuality is not something that befalls us at puberty or awakens us in early adulthood. Body play and exploration of the genitals is normal, healthy behavior on the part of the infant, toddler, and growing child. As a child is permitted normal exploration of the form and functioning of all parts of the body, the child is growing up with the acceptance of his/her sexuality from childhood on. Therefore, the need to relearn the normalcy of sexuality in adulthood decreases.

As birth is sexual, a healthy psychosexual development permits a woman greater access to her body in pregnancy and birth. For the fetus, sexuality begins when the sperm and egg merge during sexual lovemaking. The sensuality of the interuterine experience is accepted.[3] Sexual expression in birth becomes a reality as the culmination of pregnancy yields to separation of mother from baby on a biological cellular level. The normal journey through the vagina in birth is the emergence outwards of the phenomenon of conception which took that same pathway inwards to the womb during sexual intercourse. For the fetus, the interuterine experience of sexual activity throughout pregnancy may also be recognized, perhaps experienced as a physically exciting, rocking motion on the inside.

As infants discover their feet and hands, they also discover their genitals. A natural part of existence, sexuality opens us, connects us in some important way to our loving, lovable, and sensual body form. There is no beginning and no end in this view, but only the sexual cycle expressed in physical experience of ourselves and others.

REFERENCES

1. Gadpaille, W. *Cycles of Sex*. New York, Charles Scribner and Sons, 1975, pp 388-390.

2. Peterson, G. and Mehl, L. Children at Birth. *J. of Sex and Marital Therapy*, Vol. no 3, Winter, 1977.

3. Bradley, R.M., and Mistretta, C.M. Fetal Sensory Receptors, *Physiol. Rev.* 55(3): 352-382, 1975; Walker, D., Grimwade, J. and Wood, C. Intrauterine Noise: A Component of the Fetal Environment. *Am. J. Ob. Gyn.* 109(1): 91-115, 1971.; Mistretta, C.M. and Bradley, R.M. Taste and Swallowing in Utero: A Discussion of Fetal Sensory Function. *Brit. Med. Bull.* 31(1) 80-84, 1975.; Bradley, R.M. and Mistretta, C.M. Investigations of Taste Functioning and Swallowing in Fetal Sheep. In Bosma, J.F. (ed.) *Fourth Symposium on Oral Sensation and Perception.* Development in the Fetus and Infant, DHEW Publ no. (NIH) 73-546, 1975, see also the work of David Cheek and Helen Wambach.

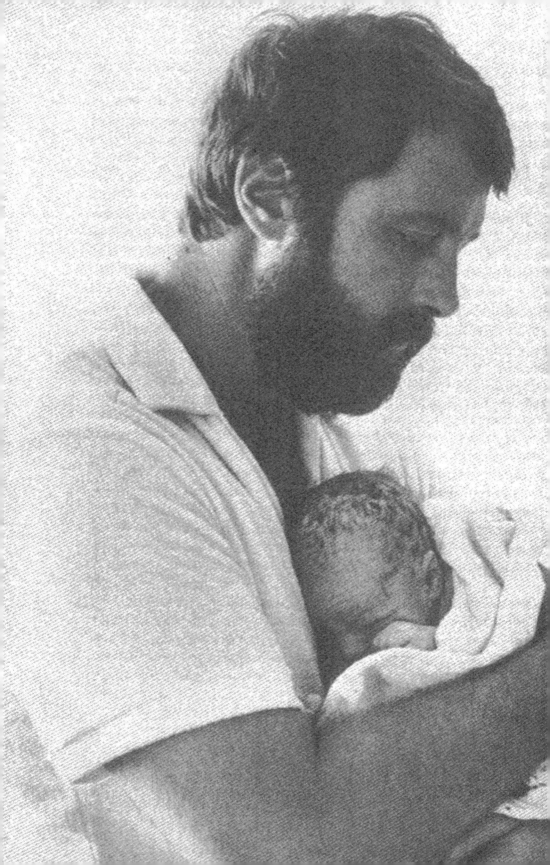

Chapter Eleven

Addressing Complications of Birth in the Prenatal Setting

Medical Model Myopia

THE DECREASE IN trust in the medical profession has sent consumers of health care scrambling to the medical texts to find their own answers. Ironically the answers sought are no more reassuring in the textbooks than they are from health care providers. Pregnant women are desiring information about the childbirth process including medical procedures and potential complications of delivery so that they may make "educated" choices regarding delivery and prepare themselves for any number of possible outcomes. Childbirth educators often find themselves in the role of information-giving and may be the persons to whom women turn for guidance in preparing for birth preparation and delivery. But what kind of an "education" are we offering women?

The "information" presented in childbirth classes arises out of the current medical model, a model increasingly distrusted by today's health care consumers. An examination of the manner in which information on complications of birth is communicated can help us to understand how such information may affect the individual woman.

The information on birth complications which is often presented in childbirth classes may not be informative in an objective sense. "Facts" are often presented with the implicit and total acceptance in randomness and physical cause and effect concepts integral to the medical model. For example, no information on the natural and healthy resolution of a complication is usually presented in preparation for childbirth. Descriptions of complications are followed by descriptions of the current popular medical interventions with little or no discussion of the "information" on any of the very regularly occurring spontaneous resolutions the woman's body may provide. Vaginal breech delivery or accounts of the many medically unexpected normal deliveries that do take place may not be presented in any detail. The childbirth educator may feel the need to give "information" on what is currently most popular in the local hospital setting. However, when we as childbirth educators *merely* reflect current acceptable local hospital practice or "medically based" information, we present only one of many possible truths; at best a presentation highly polarized in the direction of representing medically based beliefs and statistics as fact.

Pregnant women and childbirth educators alike turn to medical texts for answers. But why would we find any better or different answers there from those of the medical professional who is already becoming a disappointing figure to consumers? The medical model is a closed system. What already fits into medical theory is what is acknowledged. What does not fit is thrown into a slot which most traditionally medical researchers label "random chance". While causal relationships are examined closely in those relatively narrow statistics which support current medical theory, the large numbers in the "random chance" or "spontaneous recovery" categories are so markedly and notoriously ignored and unexamined for factors related to healthy outcome that such healthy resolutions are not included in medical statistics.

Many medical researchers have indeed become myopic as have many of our medical professionals. Healthy outcome and natural resolution of health problems have not been studied in depth as cure is believed to be a result of technology. Research has failed to look beyond the problem. We have failed to study health. We do not know the course of cure or how to promote it. This was not the case in time past. Medical doctors who practiced before technology became the god of medicine (pre-World War II) often described themselves as "helpers" to the healing process, but never as "healers". Nature, perhaps God, and the patient were recognized as the true healers. Cure was recognized and believable. The natural course of cure could be followed rather than denied.

An example of such medical model myopia is evident in the care received by several women who attended a particular prenatal clinic for their first pregnancies. Integral to the prenatal care these women received was a holistic program aimed at giving them the maximal opportunity for the birth experience desired. The community clinic where they had received holistically oriented prenatal care closed. These women received prenatal care for their second pregnancies from other doctors and midwives who depended upon the physical aspects of a woman's first birth to predict normal delivery in a second physically healthy pregnancy. The women were seen as needing no particular help during their second pregnancies, since their first births had been physiologically normal. Their medical practitioners were surprised when these women had complicated second births. The medical model did not take into account the helping energy and emotional work involved in the prenatal care that was inseparable from that first normal birth.

A biased medical orientation results when the habitual patterns of thinking in which we may have been trained leaves us "myopic" or near-sighted to the insights other fields or disciplines can offer. When little or no recognition is given to the impact of an extensive prenatal counselling program as part of the past care, the observed history of that first delivery cannot be completely understood. It simply did not occur to the medical practitioners delivering prenatal care to these women to evaluate emotional factors previously present and dealt with at the time of the first childbirth. It also did not occur to the medical care provider to attribute any significance to the emotional ambivalence (and guilt) that these individual women were struggling with in their second unplanned and unwanted pregnancies. The practitioners put all of their faith in medical statistics which reflect second births to be more predictably normal following an uncomplicated first birth experience. In this way, they became myopic to these women as individuals. Medically trained professionals making prenatal referral to counsellors may evaluate the final outcomes on purely physical grounds as they have been trained to do. They may forget to ask about the woman's feelings about her current pregnancy because her first one went smoothly from a physical perspective. Physical outcome does in fact, reflect a natural screening process for emotional issues when counselling has *not* been a part of the prenatal course. Had these women not had opportunity to explore their feelings and experience support for the emotional work coming through their first pregnancies, they indeed might have had more difficulty delivering their first babies. If the first births reflected physical complications the over-confidence of the medical practitioners would not have ensued. However the fact that each of these women reported fears that the second baby was coming too soon, *but* had a medical history of normal delivery with their first babies yielded the suggestion and encouragement from their midwives to deliver at home the second time. Traditional medical statistics do not differentiate those women receiving prenatal counselling from those who do not. The effects of counselling on the first pregnancy and the absence of counselling in a second pregnancy (about which the mothers expressed much ambivalence) are not factors for consideration in the medically trained when physical factors so prominently favor a low-risk label. These midwives were very surprised when the second birth was complicated.

As we open our hearts to new learnings, we must also open our minds to comprehend the impact of psycho-emotional integration and change within the human body. We must challenge ourselves to think along holistic lines and to experience each woman and each pregnancy as unique and individual. If we allow ourselves to experience meaning in all that occurs, we can understand what contributes to normal, healthy outcome as well as absorb a deeper comprehension of complications in birth.

Statistics: Fact or Reflection

Childbirth educators often use medical statistics and current medical texts as primary reference sources for teaching. Many childbirth educators may be offering indoctrination into the medical belief system rather than information. Possible complications of delivery need to be addressed. However the manner in which they are addressed is most important.

We are all familiar with learning situations in our lives which can be presented differently with differing effects. We may observe how a particular teacher in a daycare or school setting successfully involves the child in a particular learning task, while another teacher is unable to elicit the same enthusiasm and confidence for identical subject matter. *How* the teacher communicates affects learning.

In teaching children and adults how to swim, for example, the first item of concern addressed by the experienced teacher is the issue of confidence. The instructor knows this and does not begin the swimming lesson with information about the many possible ways to drown and the various techniques for rescue and resuscitation. He or she addresses *not drowning* by dealing with familiarity and confidence in the bodily processes for swimming. Techniques for bobbing in the water, blowing air, and floating are taught while reframing the process of drowning as even difficult. Some instructors build initial confidence in children for swimming by telling them that drowning is not easy, and that, given the techniques they are learning, drowning would be most difficult unless they panic and do not use the techniques learned. In this early phase of teaching the child to swim, very effective swimming instructors may subtly reframe "drowning" as something you must work to do. As swimming skills are mastered children may learn how to rescue and be rescued in the case of threatened drowning. The instructor *does not* interrupt the initial confidence building by diverging into probabilities of drowning and procedures that are done in the case of such a complication. Instead the experienced instructor directs and takes charge of his/her class content in order to majorly focus on confidence building, familiarity with, and techniques to aid the normal process of swimming before discussing the complications of possible drowning. If a particular student is anxious about drowning the instructor may assure the beginning swimmer that issues concerning recovery and rescue in the case of drowning will be answered and demonstrated in a future class. The instructor does not presume to attempt teaching someone who has not yet learned the techniques of swimming to learn the procedures of rescue in any detail. Nor does the swimming teacher describe in lucid detail the experience of drowning or give probabilities of it based on statistics and the number of people in the class, including a statement such as "One of you in this class will drown."; not unlike some childbirth classes in which the teacher begins or ends the class with the statement, "Three of you will have a Cesarean birth.".

In the teaching situation, such use of statistics is a distortion at best and a falsehood at worst as three people in a particular class will not necessarily have a Cesarean birth. Such communication is an improper use of medical statistics in individual application and is neither scientifically valid not emotionally useful. It serves to disrupt emotional preparation for labor and casts the woman into the emotional experience of victim before she has even begun her own individual journey into labor. Medical statistics at best reflect current trends and transitions in present day society. Self-selection factors go unrecognized for their influence on statistics. Consequently, statements taken from medical statistics communicate a static state of society. Obviously, this is not the case. Our society is in constant flux. Change in women's roles reverberates throughout the culture, affecting medical statistics.

For example, women having their first babies after the age of 35 have previously had statistically higher complications in childbearing. However, as more women are having their first babies later in the childbearing cycle of life, cultural beliefs and attitudes are changing. These women are becoming a part of a growing community and complications begin to lessen with increased opportunity for emotional expression of this group of women. Medical statistics will eventually reflect the changes in cultural as well as individual beliefs about mothering at a later age.

The childbirth professional must keep in mind that medical statistics are not static. It is a distortion of communication to present medical statistics as fact. Statistics must include a context of place, time, and the socio-cultural beliefs of the population studied to have meaning for the individual. Medical statistics make the most sense within an anthropological context. Trends and beliefs can be identified and the individual is not left without a context for human experience and understanding. Without a human context, a woman is left with only an object-orientation. To apply statistics to herself a woman must depersonalize her own experience. Depersonalization (in communication, as well as in medical practice) can only lead to alienation. A woman is robbed of her individuality when she becomes (in her own mind or in someone else's) a statistic. She becomes a victim. The experience of participating in childbirth classes should not be one of victimization. The learning experience is determined to some extent by the nature of communication or how the content of the classes is presented.

In teaching deep sea diving the expectation for normal functioning of the diving equipment is maintained even though precautions for faulty mechanisms are addressed. It is helpful to take the swimming metaphor one step further to address the extremely anxious and fearful beginning swimmer who may actually be afraid of dying by drowning. In this case it would be necessary, perhaps on an individual level, to address the issue of dying and facing that possibility before getting into the water. In the prenatal setting issues of death and dying are rarely discussed or even mildly confronted, although much time describing procedures of intervention may be spent with little or no allayance of an underlying fear of disaster.

It is common knowledge that stimulating confidence in one's

students for the ability to cope with the task at hand greatly increases the likelihood of learning the needed skills to achieve the desired process. Childbirth preparation which emphasizes coping skills and techniques for natural childbirth, is no exception. The childbirth professional can benefit greatly from the field of education on *how* to teach (including educational psychology on how to motivate) rather than looking to medicine as the prime information source. The impact of attitude and belief on the process of learning is well accepted in the fields of education, psychology, and increasingly so in the world of physical sports. Beliefs and attitudes are known to affect physical performance of athletes and dancers alike. The athlete and the dancer must cope and adjust to body workings. Feelings of confidence affect these body adjustments differently than do attitudes of dejection.

A class in deep sea diving does not digress into statistics of the possibilities of the dive being interrupted by a shark or to the extreme of quoting statistics of complications involving sharks in underwater diving. Nor does such teaching emphasize that the student should actually prepare to be such a statistic, since a certain number of people in the class will most certainly find themselves in just such a complicated situation. Instead, precautions are taught usually following a phrase "if you find yourself in the presence of a shark", or "if you see a shark coming towards you", followed by the most effective safety precaution for the situation or preparations for dealing with this circumstance. In this manner learning is specific to the situation described. Confusion results if the normal and safe situation is not described fully before turning attention to possible complications. A woman's understanding and preparation for the normal process may be neglected because of the emotional distraction which results from a digression into complication. The emotional distraction competes with the attention to the normal and safe situation when presented in close proximity or association.

The issue is one of timing and congruent communication. Many women are being asked to prepare for Cesarean birth and other complications before they even have a clear idea of what the progression of labor is when it occurs normally without complication. Women are often left with a clearer image of the possible complications of labor than of normal birth. Is it such a wonder that the complication rate is so high? If women are to prepare for normal birth, then they must be given the opportunity to do so. Preparation for possible complications should be addressed but need not precede a *thorough* presentation of the normal delivery process.

The problem of timing and congruent communication occurs in the prenatal care setting in a variety of other forms. One pregnant woman called me after having gone to a local medical facility for a pregnancy test and examination. Her doctor informed her that she was very probably pregnant as indicated by physical examination, but that she should be aware of ectopic pregnancy. Her uterus was enlarged. Her Fallopian tubes were not enlarged and were not tender. Nevertheless, she was told in detail about the operation of the Fallopian tube, should there be an ectopic pregnancy, She was sent home with instructions to call for any pain in her pelvis because her urine pregnancy test was not yet positive. The woman experienced twinges in her lower abdomen, and after considerable worry, learned from another source that normal round ligament pains could also occur during pregnancy. This woman showing a normal pregnancy was instructed to prepare for an ectopic one. As she translated these instructions into her experience she became confused. She began to distrust her normal body functioning. She was *not told what to expect if her situation was entirely normal,* which in fact it was. Her physician described in full detail the experience of ectopic pregnancy but only lightly glossed over the normal experience. It became difficult for her to learn or ascertain what was normal as the abnormal was more completely and thoroughly described to her than the normal and much more probable diagnosis. The doctor had given *specific* information in an *undefined* framework of experience. His instruction was not only misleading but anxiety-producing in the general context of pregnancy. The medical doctor may be quite aware of the normal process. However he or she may emphasize the abnormal in communication out of a caring, if not understanding concern for the patient's welfare. Communication skills are not a part of medical training, and unfortunately confusion and lack of clarity can result.

Likewise, the childbirth educator may also inadequately define the context for the information she is presenting. She may unknowingly digress in the midst of presenting the normal delivery experience to answer questions of a particular woman or couple who are expressing great concern or anxiety about complications. In attempting to be responsive to the needs of her students the childbirth educator does not take notice of the story or visualization of the normal birthing process which has been interrupted for a series of lengthy "commercials" about complicated birth. Divergent outcomes of forceps delivery, Cesarean delivery, shoulder dystocia, etc., may be experienced with some anxiety throughout the childbirth educator's reassuring description of the normal delivery patterns. The result is a confused, or double message received by the pregnant woman. Unless she *already has clear and firm beliefs about the natural safety of birth, and confidence in her own body process,* she may become confused about the safety or normalcy of the birthing process, *in general.*

Stories about women having problems, including abnormal fetal descent or position, resolved *without* medical intervention are rarely offered. The communication is that, if a problem should present itself, the *only* manner of resolution is by physical intervention. The communication may imply that the woman has no resources for resolution or adaptation to birth normally without such intervention. Incongruent communication in the class or prenatal setting can undermine the attitudes of confidence and self-reliance so important in effective teaching in any learning context.

Effective Communication

How information on complication is presented can affect the qualities of confidence and self-reliance (the very basic belief of the woman that she can give birth) *so facilitative* to the birth process and to everything else we do. Such qualities are not usually recognized by the medically trained as significant. My own clinical experience and research show the importance of confidence, self-reliance, and an internal locus of control as factors highly correlated and significantly predictive of the normal birthing process.[1-5]

Basic, effective, congruent *communication* is what is so often lacking in the prenatal care setting. Effective communication is not taught in medical or nurse midwifery schools. Nor is it taught in depth in most childbirth educator's training seminars. It is taught in some psychotherapy training programs where *how* a client expresses him/her self is the key to understanding the client's individual experiences and needs. How effectively the therapist communicates can offer the key to change in pre-set or pre-organized experience.

Women most in need of self-confidence in the birthing process are the most vulnerable to incongruent communication in childbirth classes. Women already fearful or afraid have pre-set expectations for childbirth to be complicated.

If the material taught women in childbirth classes is not congruently organized in its presentation, the teacher does not promote confidence for birthing in those women who most need it. Any woman already possessing this confidence cannot be harmed because she already has a structure of perception from which to organize the material, and may process it through her organization of experience by already presupposing confidence in herself to give birth. The woman who is *not* confident in her own ability to give birth and who has come to classes to increase her confidence in her ability to deal with labor and birth, however, may not be helped. Her confidence may remain basically unchanged, She may simply not gain in confidence for birth. Her emotional preparation or pre-organization of attitudes toward childbirth may remain the same as it was previous to her prenatal classes.

Communication does not hold the power of destruction. Nor is it endowed with "magical" powers of control or manipulation. Conscious communication can however, prove a more effective means of teaching women about birth, than can unconscious communication.

A lack of confidence and self-reliance increases the probability of a fear response to stress. When labor becomes "stressful" (as it may when women are unprepared for pain in labor), fear is a natural response. A woman may become frightened as she does not believe in her capability to adapt to the unexpected — whether it be a normal or complicated labor. The fear response is highly correlated with a decrease in oxytocin[6] and overall change in hormonal balance. The limbic system of the brain is meant to respond to the emotional context of any situation. This is its function — to modify the body's metabolism for best results in the particular situation at hand. It makes sense that fear is interpreted by the body as danger, and a common response is a decrease in the firing of oxytocin, as it would give the mother a chance to run (fight/flight response) from the dangerous situation to one safer in which to proceed with labor. In the context of sudden fear or danger during second stage labor, the ejection response is often catalyzed, (sudden release in the lower uterine segment) ensuring a fast delivery which would enable the woman to take leave of a dangerous environment.

What happens when the modern day woman's fear is the fear of birth itself? Whatever the reasons for the fear, her confidence in following through labor and birth may be mitigated. She cannot run from the part of her that harbors these fears, and uterine inertia is treated with intervention. She can make use of the available drugs or anesthesia on hand to blot out the fear. This can be a very viable alternative if the woman does not desire a natural, conscious birth process as a part of her life experience. If she does value her own conscious participation in the process (as this is one of the reasons many women attend natural childbirth classes) this may not be her preferred choice. Communication that increases confidence in a woman's ability to develop her own resources for labor offers a choice of response beyond fear for coping with whatever unknowns her labor will bring.

Congruent Communication in the Class Setting

To organize childbirth preparation material into a congruent presentation the childbirth educator needs to feel comfortable being in control of the class content. An ineffective communicator diverges for each and every question of any student at any moment. In the workshops and seminars that I teach I encourage professionals to present the course of the normal labor and delivery without interruption and as the first material to be presented. Visualization after a relaxation induction can be a very effective manner of congruent presentation of the normal delivery process although it is not the only effective method. If other methods are used in presenting this first piece of information, and questions of abnormality are raised, the educator may choose to:

1) refer the question to the question-and-answer period at the end of the presentation of the normal progression of labor,
2) refer the question to be covered during future class time on abnormal presentations, or
3) briefly answer, but not digress from, and return to, the *normal* birthing process.

This is the usual format in most educational settings. The normal process is given full attention before more complex material is presented. It is during this first initial and complete presentation that the message of birth as a normal, safe, and natural process can be communicated to the audience. A congruent communication is one in which all sensory channels (hearing, seeing, feeling) are in agreement with the message. The pregnant woman can indulge in the visual image as well as in the feeling of the words as she hears the childbirth educator describe the normal birthing experience. After this material is complete, further information on complications and abnormal procedures can take place *without competing* with the initial presentation of normal birth. People learn by processing information given in such a way as to represent its application on a personal level. A complete and full sensory explanation of normal birth enables the pregnant woman to represent to herself an experience of normal delivery. The information has been communicated congruently if the pregnant woman is able to represent to herself an internal experience of the natural process. Use of visualization for childbirth preparation may provide women with the opportunity to experience an internal representation of the normal birthing process on a personal level.

Addressing Complications in Childbirth Classes

One of the commonest means of effectively presenting complication material is to present it in a special class set aside just for such discussion. This is particularly helpful if the childbirth educator is willing to schedule extra time for a "fear session" specifically about fears in childbirth. Clear descriptions of complications and needed discussion of information available on the topic of abnormal birthing can occur. Complications can then be discussed in full and in detail without competing with the learnings of the normal delivery process. A separate class may even be set aside for Cesarean birth. There is a place and time for every concern. Childbirth educators may benefit from observing how much time is spent on the normal as well as abnormal delivery patterns in class content.

In one of my workshops on Holistic Prenatal Care, a childbirth educator explored how she had responded to the needs of one particularly anxious women in the classes who had experienced a previous Cesarean. The woman was planning for a vaginal delivery with her second child. She needed special attention, which she received in the classes as she was very vocal about her fears and anxieties. Much time was spent on the detail of the Cesarean birth experience and the woman's plans for it, in the case that she needed a second operation. She was able to work through her own anxieties of her Cesarean experience. However, approximately 70 percent of the time spent on the birth process in the classes was used for description of Cesarean birth and the various complications leading to the operation. The childbirth educator discovered that in fact, normal delivery was not given equal time, nor time for uninterrupted presentation and involvement. The woman had a vaginal delivery after her previous Cesarean. Out of 7 women in the class 5 women (all primigravidae) had Cesareans.

The vocal woman had worked through her own anxiety in the class setting; however, her experience of Cesarean birth may have pre-empted the time needed for other members of the class to experience and prepare for the normal process. The childbirth educator found herself to be out of control of class content and process, as she felt compelled to respond to the most vocal person and thereby tailored the class to the needs of one woman. Consequently, the class members were guided by the needs and concerns of one woman who had experienced Cesarean birth and *not* by the needs and concerns of adapting to the challenges and/or difficulties of a normal delivery. In retrospect, it became apparent to the childbirth educator that the woman preparing for a vaginal delivery after Cesarean may have special needs which could be addressed individually.

It is, of course, unknown whether spending more time on normal birthing (which would have enabled the women having Cesareans to spend more time on coping skills for normal delivery) would have affected the physiology of their birthing processes. Perhaps an equal amount of time spent on normal and abnormal birthing patterns would have yielded the same results. Perhaps not. For women already lacking confidence in the birthing process, it may have *helped* to have addressed normal birthing to a greater extent. However by no means am I suggesting that these women were *harmed* by a lessened focus on the normal. But perhaps the outcomes were *unchanged* for the women already afraid and lacking confidence in the birthing process. As a therapist, I am most interested in catalyzing change. Midwives, childbirth educators, and physicians can be both sensitive and influential. It may be fruitful for the childbirth educator as well as for the midwife and physician to contemplate the potential for serving as a change agent in the prenatal setting.

Normal birthing does require adaptation, especially for the primigravida. Too often, class time spent on adjusting to normal birthing and dealing with the pain of labor does *not* get as much time as presentation and discussion of complications of childbirth. One study done on primigravidae[7] showed a negative correlation between childbirth education and normal delivery. What are we teaching women? Perhaps in *some* situations these women would be better off left untaught. This last statement is not necessarily my belief, but is meant to stimulate thought regarding how we "prepare" women for birth. We cannot prepare women for childbirth. We can only help women to ready themselves to meet the unknown in themselves during the labor process, as they meet with nature to give birth to the beauty of physical human form. If we can deal with fears of the unknown in the normal process, such as dealing with pain of labor and with our self-images as pregnant women giving birth to ourselves in motherhood and in family-hood, then we can stimulate resources for dealing with any situation. To interrupt the presentation of normal delivery with presentation of abnormal labor patterns prevents women from dealing with the anxieties, concerns, and fears about the *normal* process. Anxieties and fears are too often only discussed as relevant to the abnormal delivery. Normal delivery fears and concerns get little attention and so may not have opportunity to be worked through. There is a tendency also, for fears and anxieties about the abnormal situation to be more externally focused. Fears and anxieties associated with normal delivery often yield an internal focus on adjustment to belief and attitude change.

Through my work with pregnant women, I have learned from them that any of the fears, concerns, and feelings that come up in a complicated birth can come up, and do occur, in the normal labor and delivery. By addressing anxieties of complication only, it is as if we communicate that, should these feelings come up, they are connected with abnormal as opposed to normal birthing. This in itself can precipitate fear in labor. Very often women report that because they did not talk about pain in their childbirth classes, when they experienced pain in hard labor they were very sure that "something was going wrong" in their bodies. They had been taught that normal delivery did not hurt if certain breathing mechanisms were employed and if intellectually they knew what was going on.

Knowing what is going on in the body can facilitate coping with the experience of pain whether it be childbirth, abortion, or any other process. So can relaxation and breathing facilitate coping. It does not mean that knowing these things *prevents* the experience of pain. Obstetrics and childbirth education have often fallen short of dealing with the natural and healthy emotional stress generated in pregnancy and labor.

A knowledge of complications can facilitate coping with anxiety, should complications occur, but does not necessarily prevent the occurrence of anxiety. Knowledge of normal delivery can be just as important in dealing with anxieties about pain in labor, though it will not necessarily prevent pain from occuring. Dealing with anxieties and fears about the abnormal birthing process can help prepare a woman for dealing with complicated birth. It *does not* however, necessarily prepare a woman for dealing with *un*complicated birth. Childbirth classes seem to have strayed further and further from adequately dealing with the reality of normal birthing.

Normal Fears and Their Expression

If a woman expresses fears and anxieties that are considered "normal", her physician, midwife, or childbirth educator may close the door on further communication about the subject with "Oh, that's a perfectly normal reaction." While the professional is attempting to be reassuring he or she is also very definitely telling the woman that there is nothing more to discuss. The best meaning practitioners sometimes view their jobs as that of assuming the worry for their clients. Though this may be far from her intent, the practitioner's communication can reflect a behavioral attitude of discussing only the physical "problems" of birth in any detail. Constant reassurance may reflect that the practitioner is assuming too much responsibility for the woman's task of emotional preparation.

A particular midwife responded to her client's continued statements of anxiety about the baby by telling her it was a normal reaction and finally by imploring the client and her husband to let her (the midwife) do the worrying for them, since she was paid to do so. The midwife refused to observe this as an emotional issue needing further attention because it was "normal" to have such fears. She felt her job was to reassure the pregnant woman and in this way take care of her. The woman gave birth to a stillborn. The midwife could not be paid to grieve for her, just as she could not in actuality "worry" for her. The woman's attempt to worry about her baby can be understood as a natural need. In this case, her worry may have helped prepare her for dealing with future loss. She was, in fact, not "surprised" by the outcome, although she was in grieving for her loss. As practitioners we cannot take the emotionality out of pregnancy, birth, or life; be it joy or sorrow, worry or pain. We cannot feel *for* our clients. We can only feel *with* them.

The work of "worrying" can serve an emotional purpose of working through feelings and attitudes that are held at abeyance because of fear. When a woman is very worried about having a particular outcome (stillbirth, genetic or other defect) I often ask her to go further into her fear. I might ask her to imagine the occurrence most feared, and how she would deal with it. It is usually very common for a change in attitude to take place after allowing herself to think about the "unthinkable". Worrying may signal emotional work not being recognized that needs attention. The practioner can facilitate a deepening of resources and coping capacity in the individual woman by being unafraid him/herself to address the fear on an emotionally direct level. In this way, the practitioner can be *with* the woman. She is not alone. Well-intended medical professionals often do not easily tolerate communications of an emotional nature, unless they are extreme and considered "abnormal". They may not understand the "work of worrying" as the possible emotional work of the pregnant woman in preparation for the unknown of birth in a modern society.

Medical professionals and childbirth educators alike are not usually trained to deal with emotions and feelings. Medicine teaches facts and statistics. *Therefore, in order for a pregnant woman to gain the attention to emotional issues she may need,* she very often resorts to fantasies of the abnormal situation. She may continually request that the professional talk with her about what would happen *if something went wrong.* If she cannot gain rapport and discussion of her feelings by talking about them in context of the normal delivery, she often resorts to concentration on complicated delivery in order to address the very real fears and feelings of the normal process. In this manner, a woman's behavior is often shaped towards dealing with abnormal delivery and not normal delivery. Anything defined as "normal" (be it emotional or physical) may not be *thoroughly* and adequately discussed, described, or concentrated upon, as is the abnormal. It may be important to address that which is defined as "normal" with as much concentration to detail as is often the case for the "abnormal".

The growing percentage of time spent on abnormal birthing in natural childbirth classes *mirrors* this concentration on the abnormal by medically trained professionals. We are already aware of the impact of the traditional medical orientation in obstetrics in this country. Childbirth education can learn from the mistakes of the traditional medical model and its neglect of the consideration of and interest in the normal delivery. If we can begin to study what goes well and why, instead of only what goes wrong and why, we begin to embark upon a holistic understanding of birth. What contributes to birthing when all goes well needs to be explored as thoroughly and perhaps even more thoroughly than abnormal birth.

Women requiring more time on complications for whatever reasons (past experience, anxiety, etc.) can be adequately accommodated, and perhaps more appropriately so, on an individual basis. Private sessions can augment the general series of classes. Preoccupation with complication definitely needs to be addressed for the individual on a group basis. However if it persists, such preoccupation can be understood as a special request for help and may be addressed on an individual level. Excessive preoccupation with complications need not pre-empt the time needed to thoroughly address the normal process in a group setting.

"Birth Trauma" — A Misinterpretation

As many of the new "birth psychologies" of the last decade have entered the American scene, confirming birth as a normal and healthy process has become increasingly necessary. Primal scream, rebirthings, and regressions to traumatic experience of birth have led some people into the misguided conception that all birth is traumatic[8-9]. These beliefs, as well as those promulgated by the medical profession about birth have burdened women with a concept that is ungrounded in physiology. The belief that birth is an inherently traumatic event bridles women with the concept of a labor that in some manner is hurting her baby. Although untrue from a purely biological perspective of normal birth, trauma has been experienced biologically and perhaps psychologically in the past two generations of technological birth.

Belief in birth as traumatic became popular as some psychologists and psychiatrists "regressed" clients back to the experience of their own births. However two important factors have been overlooked in the hasty proclamation of birth as traumatic. These are:

1.) that in the past two generations, birth has been abnor-

mally traumatic and intervened with, especially in terms of prolonged nursery isolation of newborns as routine,
2.) that these "regressions" are influenced by feelings regarding the present day relationship between the person being regressed and his/her mother.

It is impossible to have a true "regression", that is, a state that is purely representative of a past experience as we are never without the experiences and resources of our lives since that experience. "Regressions" can only reconstruct that which occurred in the past, *filtered through* influences of our present. We cannot totally separate our present and subsequent life experience and personhood, from that which came before.

"Regressions" to past birth experiences have been done with a pre-selected group (the past two generations) experiencing the routine trauma of childbirth intervention and/or early separation. We must not mistake the birth trauma of the last two generations as normal or natural to the birthing process. Though early separation of newborn from an anesthetized mother was routine in the past generation or two in this country (as well as forceps delivery and other birth technology), does not mean that birth is traumatic. Rather, it is the case that the average birth taking place in the past generation is traumatic. Problematic delivery is traumatic. Forceps, especially high forceps (so much more common in obstetrical practice in the late 40's and early 50's) can be traumatic. Early separation and nursery isolation after birth can be traumatic.

Naturally, if we "regress" ourselves to our births, most of us will experience some problem or trauma associated with birth technology and/or the routine hospital procedures of the 1950's and earlier. However, to deduce from such "regressions" that birth itself is traumatic, or that *all* births are traumatic is a short-sighted conclusion. Therapists espousing the belief in birth as traumatic for the baby draw their conclusions from "regressions" of their clients, (many of them experiencing problematic births). They do not draw their conclusions from first hand knowledge or experience of being present at the healthy deliveries of babies born without complication or difficulty. Those of us who have been present at the births of babies born without problems or complications of birth find it very difficult to imagine the experience of such babies to be "traumatic". Wonder, surprise, and adjustment to external warmth and love seem apparent, but in no way do these babies appear "traumatized".

In addition to the very probable trauma of birth found in the generation now of childbearing age, is also the very natural influence of present day feelings for the mothers of our own "regressive" experiences.

It can prove very helpful to an individual woman to explore the experience of her own birth. In the case in which she finds it particularly negative, whatever the reasons, it can be very beneficial to engage a woman in a re-working of that experience, in her own birth visualization, or "re-birthing". Indeed, many of the complications of birth experienced by women today may have an association to their own alienation in birth. This may be particularly true of women who have been born prematurely themselves, and experienced prolonged separation following birth with very little human contact. However it complicates a woman's preparation for birth to insist that birth itself is traumatic, rather than that specific problematic birth can be traumatic. Women also very often spontaneously work through their own traumatic experiences of birth long before they ever become pregnant, oftentimes within the context of a loving mother-daughter relationship.

A belief in birth as inherently traumatic is disrespectful of the naturally healthy and very normal process of birth. Women desiring a normal and natural process of labor and birth are burdened by a false premise that such a birth, regardless of its normalcy (and seeming ease to the baby as it is born) will be hurtful, and "difficult" for the baby. A woman is being asked to give birth naturally on the one hand, but warned of the inevitable "trauma" to her baby that her body will be doing in labor! What loving mother would not secretly prefer a Cesarean, given this belief? The belief in birth as traumatic parallels the medical belief in birth as difficult and risky.

As women, we are in a position of reclaiming our rights to nature. In a society that has strayed from a biological definition of normalcy to a sociological one, a return to trust in nature is essential if we are to begin our return to normal birth[10].

Blame: The By-Product of Ignorance

Qualities of confidence and self-reliance consist of personal attitudes and beliefs that have impact on the childbearing process. However many medical professionals project the concern that addressing the effects of attitudes and beliefs is to "blame". It is as if the medical field itself has lost its belief in the human resource of compassion in the clinical setting. The resources for understanding human belief systems are not recognized, and yet are sorely needed knowledge for the medical practitioner. The medical professional often seems to fear his/her own inability to deal empathically with the emotional aspects of beliefs and attitudes in the health care setting. Yet, women respond to emotional as well as technological support. There is no need for us to deny that which is necessary, helpful and supportive to the process of labor through technology. It is also unnecessary for us to remain ignorant of the natural existence and need for the emotional work of pregnancy and birth in preparing for motherhood, especially in our times of stress in the cultural redefinition of family.

Modern woman is questing for integration of her role as mother, lover, wife, and often works outside as well as inside the home. The natural and healthy stress of pregnancy has heightened as we work through our changing times. Women deserve respect and recognition for the emotional work of pregnancy, the task of identity integration that is inevitable as she crosses the threshold of motherhood. It should be no surprise to us that this period of natural stress has become for many women, distressful, as the work of integration goes unrecognized. Within a holistic model, opportunity for free expression of concerns must be offered. It is through such freedom of expression that women may integrate their feelings and change beliefs and attitudes that bind them in their journey.

As a mental health professional, I am aware through my training and experience that beliefs and attitudes about our bodies and the world stem first from our original family's belief system and secondarily from our environment and cultural heritage. It is not necessary to blame in order to recognize and address the impact of a person's attitudes and beliefs on physical process, any more than a medically trained professional (nor I) would appropriate blame to the individual who inherited a genetic disease or abnormality. It does not occur to me to blame a person for his or her family's beliefs and cultural influence. It is also illogical to grant total control of body functioning to beliefs and attitudes, but rather to acknowledge the impact on physical functioning that attitudes and emotions generate. We cannot expect people to be any more in control of their emotions than they are of their bodies. Control comes only in action. It is an illusion to believe we can control our minds any more than our bodies. Our behavior and our actions are all that we control.

If we find ourselves feeling angry, for example, or sad, we

cannot make ourselves *not* feel that which we are feeling at the moment. Our control as human beings comes through our behavioral interpretation of that feeling but not in the control of the experience of feeling. We can control our actions when we are angry. We can control our behavioral response so as not to physically abuse anyone through the expression of such anger. We can control ourselves to not behaviorally physicalize sadness into suicidal behavior, by coming up with alternate means of coping with our emotionality as human beings. We cannot however, make ourselves feel differently by exercise of will or control. Only through freedom of expression to feel our emotions can we reorganize our conceptual framework of the world and our experience of ourselves within it. Beliefs change naturally as a result of exploration of feelings and values that are conflicted. Without the encouragement and support to explore our feelings and beliefs we become rigid and unyielding to the changes inherent in life.

Change is inevitable in the life process of the pregnant woman. Through the experience of feeling as process we make choices about how we take ourselves through our natural emotions during pregnancy, birth, and other life cycles. If we cannot control having feelings to begin with then how is it that we are to blame ourselves for our feelings? Feelings, attitudes, and beliefs are as naturally and organically grown as any flower that takes root in the earth's soil. Children too are grown within the necessary human elements of emotions, beliefs, and attitudes in the family that nurtures them and the cultural environment that fosters their needed societal involvement. We as women do not exist apart or alone from our culture, our families, or our homes. In pregnancy as in other life processes, we do not exist apart from our beliefs and the physical body which experiences feeling.

Compassion for ourselves as emotional as well as physical human beings will free us to explore our beliefs and attitudes and offers opportunity for change and renewed vitality throughout life. Blame is merely the by-product of innocent ignorance. Perhaps it is time we take ourselves outside of the constraints of blame so that we may free ourselves towards a further knowledge of health, or any other field in which human understanding and compassion are essential elements.

REFERENCES

1. Easton, P., Peterson, G., and Mehl, L. "Prediction of Women at Risk for Cesarean Section". In Peterson, G. and Mehl, L. *Holistic Prenatal Care*. Berkeley, Mindbody Press, in press.

2. Toney, J., McRae, J., Peterson, G., and Mehl, L. "Differences Among Women at Risk for Birth Complications." In Peterson, G. and Mehl, L. op. cit.

3. McRae, J., Peterson, G., and Mehl, L. "Discrimination of Birth Complications from Prenatal Interviews." In Peterson, G. and Mehl, L., op. cit.

4. McRae, J., Peterson, G., and Mehl, L. "Psychiatric Diagnosis, Defenses, and Anxiety in Relation to Birth Complications." In Peterson, G. and Mehl, L., op. cit.

5. Peterson, G., *Birthing Normally: A Personal Growth Approach to Childbirth,* Berkeley, Mindbody Press, 1983.

6. See Figure 1 – Fear diagram; Kelly, J. V., "Effect of Fear Upon Uterine Motility." Am. J. Obstet. Gynecol. 83(5): 576–587, March 1962; Newton, N., Foshee, D., Newton, M., "Parturient Mice: Effect of Environment on Labor." Science 151 (3717): 1560–1561, March 1966; Newton, N., Peeler, D., and Newton, M. "Effect of Disturbance on Labor." Am. J. Ob. Gyn. 101(8):1096–1102, August, 1968; Newton, N., Foshee, D., and Newton, M. "Environmental Inhibition of Labor through Environmental Disturbance." Ob. Gyn. 27(3): 371–377, March 1966; Rosenfeld, C.R. and West, J. "Circulatory Response to Systemic Infusion of Norepinephrine in the Pregnant Ewe." Am. J. Obstet. Gynecol. 127: 376–383, February, 1977; Anderson, S.G., Still, J.G., and Greiss, F.C. "Differential Reactivity of the Gravid Uterine Vasculatures: Effects of Norepinephrine." Am. J. Obstet. Gynecol. 129(3):293–298, October 1977.

7. Ettner, R. "Psychological Aspects of Uterine Inertia." In Peterson, G. and Mehl, L., op. cit.

8. Capra, Fritjof, *The Turning Point: Science, Society and the Rising Culture,* Simon and Schuster, New York, 1982. See Chapter 11 for a discussion on the work of Stanislav Grof.

9. Birth regression refers to a guided therapeutic experience involving the theoretical re-experiencing of one's own birth. See Cheek, David, B. and LeCron, Leslie, *Clinical Hypnotherapy,*

Grune and Stratton, New York, 1968, for more information on these approaches. See Schwartz, Lenny, *The World of the Unborn: Nurturing Your Child Before Birth,* Marek Publishers, New York, 1980 for a personal description of a birth regression.

10. This section was taken from *Holistic Prenatal Care.*

Section IV
Holistic Principles in Risk Screening

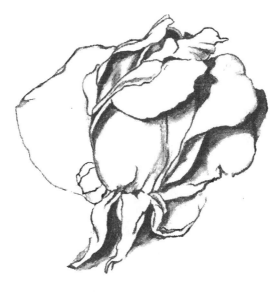

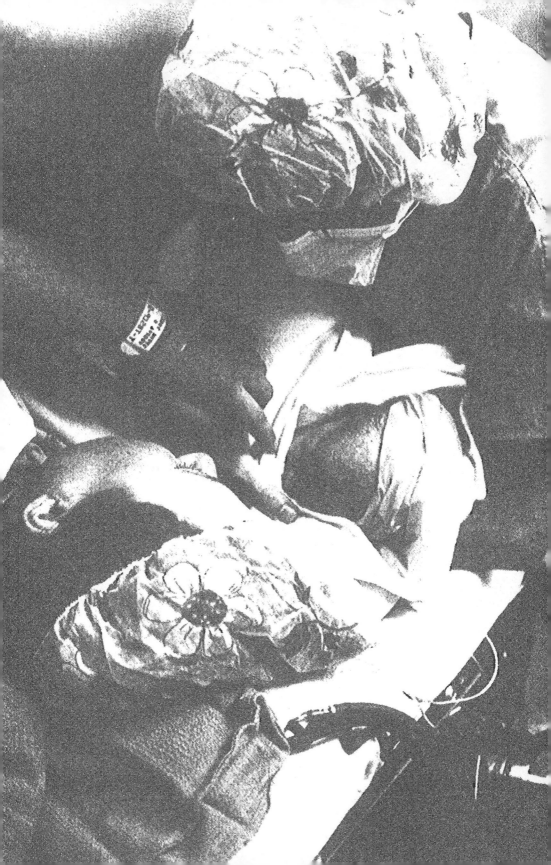

Chapter Twelve

Holistic Screening for Risk

Lewis Mehl, MD, Ph.D

THE PURPOSE OF this next chapter is to consider some of the ways the information provided in the preceding chapters can be used to aid in screening for risk. The method we will discuss is that of descriptive phenomenology. Phenomenology is a way of gaining knowledge about a person that emphasizes: 1) giving up all prior assumptions and beliefs about that person and their situation, and 2) suspending all prior judgments. Then we can make a complete narrative description of that person which can then be used to make conclusions.

Typically, psychologists believe that pregnancy can be a very stressful time, requiring adaptation to enable growth and maturation to occur, especially for women who must, for the first time, meet the challenges of pregnancy and the subsequent experience of mothering.[1,2] What they have not recognized is that these changes and the reactions to them have physiological consequences. Bibring, et al.[3] point out that pregnancy involves changes (physical and psychological) that are irreversible—the woman can never not be a mother again. Facing this fact may also have physiological consequences. This is not usually appreciated by psychologists or physicians. Usually the reason is inadequate knowledge about the person. Nadelson[4] states that a physician may perform well in the technical procedures with limited ability to respond to the psychosocial needs of the women. Some of this may be because modern obstetric practice does not allow the physician sufficient time to get to know the client on a deeper level than the superficial 5-10 minute office visit.

One way the problem of time pressure can be solved is to work with a team of other health professionals. At least one, and preferably two, members of that team should have some psychological training and sophistication. A team implies a small group which can have its own problems and dynamics that can interfere with the accurate assessment of the client.

Feelings and fears experienced during pregnancy are intense and varied.[4] Women often express concern about areas of life that had previously seemed conflict free. These include future role and responsibility, marriage and career plans, sexual relationships, and physical body image.[4-6] These concerns frequently arise during any transition. Sexual conflicts can surface during pregnancy, since pregnancy is such an obvious overt statement of sexuality.[4] Conflicts concerning the woman's early relationship with her mother and her experience of having been mothered can surface or re-appear easily during pregnancy.[7] None of these conflicts *per se* may necessarily have physiological consequences. What is meaningful is the total gestalt of conflicts, and especially how the woman resolves conflict in her life. How is her actual describable life influenced by these conflicts? What type of behavioral patterns can be seen underlying the way she attempts to resolve such conflicts. Here is where we begin to dive from the anatomical surface, to the depths of physiology. These coping patterns and styles may represent the basic biobehavioral patternings which involve the autonomic nervous system and other neurohormonal processes. Beliefs serve as anchors and guideposts to the understanding of the direction of flow of such processes.

Potential Conflict Areas

It is a fact of American society that money must be paid for medical services rendered. The exceptions to this are prepaid health care plans in which premiums are paid by the participator or his/her employer. Paying money is a stress unless one has so much money that the fee for prenatal care and delivery is perceived as miniscule. It is always somewhat of a hardship. Freud recognized this when he recommended that the client be charged an amount for psychotherapy sufficient for him or her to experience the payment as at least some type of hardship. The stress of having to pay money can expose biological patterns of response to stress. For example, an underlying biobehavioral pattern of holding tightly onto things before giving them up could be a response set to hold onto money until the last moment and then give it up with only great prodding by the practitioner. In our (Holistic Psychotherapy and Medical Group) study of the

Berkeley Family Health Center, a community clinic in Berkeley, people who exhibited difficulties in keeping payment plans they had agreed to tended to be at higher risk than people who conscientiously paid their bills according to their individual payment plan. Payment plans took into account money available. If someone didn't have much money, but conscientiously paid their bills even at a small rate, this was not associated with risk. Paying nothing might say something about their investment in the process, and their motivation for following the prenatal program effectively.

Any of the conflicts we have discussed can cause feelings of guilt, anger, ambivalence, and remorse,[4] all of which have neurohormonal and physiological consequences. In addition, the implications of pregnancy for lifestyle change are tremendous. They are enough to force anyone but the most naive toward self-reflection and consideration with perhaps some trepidation. Then the physiologically important question is how such issues are resolved in the past. The best way to determine this is to obtain a life history that includes sufficient information to identify previous crises. Then we can list everything of significance that happened after the crisis. This is done in a phenomenological way in that everything is fair game to be included. If there was an accident in the six months after a major crisis, this would be as valid as a breakdown in the functioning of the physical body.

Conflicts with parents may arise during pregnancy. This can be especially so if the grandmother-to-be begins to see the daughter as an equal and no longer as a child. Then she may produce and nourish conflict with the daughter either in a competitive sense to prove she is a better mother or because she does not want to accept the notion of ageing implied in becoming a grandmother.[7]

A woman may have had a previous abortion, about which she still feels guilty. She may begin to think more about it as the reality of pregnancy becomes apparent. This also presents a challenge that she needs to resolve. This seems all the more so if a previous child has been adopted out. Memories are often state-specific. They and the accompanying feelings may have been so much a part of the emotional state of being pregnant that memory is repressed to avoid the emotional state that it triggers. Then, when that state is entered, the woman remembers traumatic events she had previously forgotten. If she is afraid of the personal emotional consequences of facing these memories, fear can result. That fear can prevent those memories from being accessible to consciousness.

There are physiological consequences of such fear. Some of these are well-known. Fear decreases the amount of blood reaching the baby. This can cause the baby to be very susceptible to fetal distress during labor due to the chronic problem with lack of oxygen. Fear can prevent or disrupt an effective uterine contraction pattern. This physiological response to fear makes sense in the animal kingdom. An animal uses this reflex to stop labor in the presence of danger or to suddenly eject the fetus if in the late pushing stage of labor. For people, much of their fear is generated from images or thoughts rather than external events. The consequences can be just as physiological.

Relationship problems can also occur during pregnancy. A knowledge of the couple's relationship is very important for assessing risk. The couple's relationship is more powerful than either individual alone. A knowledge of the past ways a woman has responded to stress may be insufficient for accurate prediction in the present if the previous stress was not within the context of that present relationship. A woman can be very strong alone, but in the context of her relationship become very weak to allow her husband to be strong. This occurred with one woman we were acquainted with whose husband was out of the country on business. She seemed exceptionally strong and independent until he returned. Prior to his return she had been assertive and aggressive. At his return, she followed him meekly to appointments and was very quiet while he did all the talking. She seemed to recede into the background within the context of their relationship. One had to separate her ability and history of coping without him from her behavior when her husband was available. This knowledge allows a successful prediction of her risk for labor. More will be said about this later. The man may be threatened by the woman being both powerful and pregnant. He may feel angry or ambivalent because of the perceived threat the child may pose to the relationship, from feeling a need to compete with the child for the woman's love and attention, or feeling that all the woman's feelings and affections may go to the child leaving none for him.[8] It is very important to observe how these issues are handled in the context of the relationship and to be able to predict risk status for delivery.

Sexual issues can be very important during pregnancy.[4] This again presents an issue which must be coped with. There are also feelings related to the change in body image. Some women are reported as having increased feelings of dependency, passivity, and a desire to be alone.[9] Some authors believe this may be in part physiological.[4] However, the entire phenomenon is psychophysiological. Thus, the psychophysiological changes of pregnancy present another task which must be coped with.

In the remainder of this chapter, I will provide more information on some of the specific factors that can be searched for as potent factors that can begin an assessment. These factors need to be looked at as situations with which to cope and general areas from which specific beliefs that represent behavioral patterns can be extracted. This will become more clear as the material unfolds. Thus, in the example about payment behavior, money is a symbol regarding the process of exchanging something dear to someone for something else. If the client is not paying, perhaps it means "I don't trust you" or "I'm not sure about you," or "I don't want to commit myself to you or to the process." Any of these stances toward life or exchange can be part of an underlying psychophysiological pattern that will affect physiology.

Initial Interview

We recommend that contact with the client begin as an unstructured time which can be a consultation type format in which the client interviews the practitioner. In such a form they have to decide how to approach the practitioner. If they're hostile from the opening sentences, that can be a very meaningful piece of experience to integrate into the overall view of the client. In this first appointment much can be learned. Psychiatrists and psychologists have recognized many of the tumultuous changes pregnancy brings to the family and the personality. They have not appreciated how direct the impact of these processes can be on the woman's physiology.

This kind of important information is immediately accessible. In the first interview if the woman sits very quietly and still and her man does all the talking, this is a statement about their relationship. If the relationship is such that the woman has developed a coping style that the husband takes care of her problems for her, that might not be a good coping style for labor. Psychophysiologically the woman may be patterned to expect her husband (mate) to take care of stress that affects her. This expectation in labor could cause her to "psychophysiologically" be unable to maintain the force of her uterine contractions when confronted with the stress of pain. She may turn to someone else to take over.

In the initial interview in which the client is allowed to structure the time, much can be learned, including information on the couple's relationship or the people's view of themselves. People may present themselves to be taken care of or may want to be an active participant in their health care. In any practice setting, clients may have preconceived ideas about the personal attributes, values, and ideas of the health care provider. These include the belief that doctors are all avaricious, wealthy, and unfriendly or that midwives will always do what the client wants. It may take some time to realize inaccurate preconceptions. Some may never realize their preconceptions. Some may continue to be hostile and suspicious despite the best efforts of the practitioner to allay their fear. The way each client approaches the practitioner initially provides very valuable information prior to the formal history taking process. During the history, more of the practitioner's attributes are visible and a manipulative patient can easily learn the correct responses. This happened in one study case with a woman who saw herself as a witch and concealed this by learning the practitioner would not respond positively to this side of her life. This happened when she gave her religion as pagan, and he jokingly asked her if she were a witch.

History Taking

The purpose of the history taking is both to obtain a good medical data base of factors that would affect the pregnancy and to obtain contextual information regarding these events. If the woman had a severe pelvic infection, I would want to know what was happening in her life during that time. I'd want to understand what this pelvic infection was a logical expression of. If we believe as Medard Boss[10] does, that physical illness or disease states represent a "bodying forth" of some basic aspect of that person's existence, then we need a more existence-oriented profile of life around the time of the illness. Many people ask how does one have the time for that? One answer is to use a history questionnaire that covers the basic areas of a history so that time is not wasted asking questions for which there are no positive answers. Some people will admit to problems in the anonymous world they share with a pencil and paper questionnaire that they will deny within the interrelationship dynamics of interacting with another human being. Examples of such topics include sexuality, emotional problems, and alcohol and drug abuse. This is especially so since many patients in American culture see it as very negative to have emotional problems. They see a certain honor in having physical problems but are very resistant to the psychophysiological concept. This is an intriguing area. I would naively assume that the goal of the patient is the restoration of a state of health. This means coming to the doctor or practitioner in a relatively open-minded fashion and considering their answers and suggestions. This is not, of course, what usually happens. Often the patient comes with a collection of symptoms which they fear represents disease in a particular organ. They don't want to think that their problem is "all in their heads." (As if anything in physical existence could be "all in the head.") They want something to be physically wrong with them. Perhaps this is because of the Western technological ethos. People may think that Western medical technology can quickly correct their problem if it's physical. Little do they realize that most of their "physical" conditions pursue an inexorable downhill course in Western medical thought. Drugs and surgery usually only delay the inevitable, with a few exceptions. In these exceptions there can be a "cure" of the disease, yet then side effects of the treatment often occur. This is true from minor problems to major problems. The patient with a urinary tract infection who is treated with antibiotics may recover quickly from her bladder problem. Then she might experience a severe vaginal infection associated with the antibiotic killing all the normal vaginal bacteria, thereby paving the way for yeast or other pathogens, which are normally present but kept in check by the healthy bacteria, (lactobacilli) to invade the unprotected mucosa (vaginal wall). The patient who is successfully treated for Hodgkin's disease (a type of cancer) may then develop leukemia as a side effect of the medication.

Why should this be? If the faith of Western people in drugs and surgery were complete, then the response should be complete. Perhaps this faith is not so complete and in times of crisis we revert to an earlier, religiously-oriented cultural self who is suspicious of our technological gods. Perhaps this lack of total response is because illness is a "bodying forth" of disturbances in the foundations of personal existence not adequately treated by surgery or drugs. The exception to this could be the person who has spontaneously resolved their problem during the time of the illness. If a person has developed an infection associated with depression over loss of a lover and feelings of hopelessness and despair (which result in suppresion of the body's immune system) and then gets pneumonia, that person could make creative changes during this time, redefining his or her life not in terms of identity with the other, but in terms of identity with his or her own self. Then treatment can be successful because the disorder in existence has been cured. A belief in drugs and doctors can then allow for a cure without the continuation of other problems.

Physical Exam

The physical examination can serve as an important time to assess the client's relationship to her body. During the physical exam another kind of stress occurs. The sex of the examiner allows for the gathering of some additional information. It is more understandable for the woman to be somewhat shy about her body if the examiner is a man. In the context of our culture, a physical examination of a woman by a man presents some unique challenges and situations which can be colored by past experience. The possible sexual connotations of such an exam are evident as the man must feel the woman's breasts and must insert both speculum and fingers into her vagina. How the woman responds to the physical examination says something about how ensconced she is in sexual stereotypes or in response sets which are productive of dysfunctional behavior patterns (while nevertheless remaining culturally maintained). If the practitioner offers the client a chance to participate in the exam by feeling her own uterus or looking at her own cervix and this seems disgusting to the patient, that may be part of a larger behavioral pattern that needs to be considered and understood.

Some women don't want to look at their bodies and don't want to be part of the birth, but still want to have a normal, enjoyable birth experience, sometimes at home. How could this be interpreted in a biobehavioral model? Such attitudes could mean nothing, or could be part of a biobehavioral pattern with physiological consequences.

Birth is very much a body process. It is a process that seems to work best with the woman integrating her consciousness with her body, as a vine climbs a fence row. This requires qualification. If the woman has always dealt with stresses involving the physical body by dissociating her mind from the process and that has been uniformly successful in the past, such a coping syle (biobehavioral pattern) could be a good sign for a normal labor.

The belief this represents is "under stress my body works for me. All I have to do is step aside and let it." Actually among many middle to upper income Bay Area women with whom we worked, the process was reversed, These women seemed to obsess so much about their physical body processes that they needed to let their minds step outside and allow their bodies to work for them. Their belief was, "My body doesn't and won't work well unless I think and worry about it so much that it has to."

This is similar to Emir, Jane Robert's character who demands that the sky not allow any rain only to suffer the consequences of compliance with this demand.[16] Emir is sent forth in a small boat by his father, the King of a newly formed kingdom on a newly formed earth, to discover the names of things. Emir hates rain and asks, asks, asks, and finally demands that the sky stay clear. As the river on which he is travelling becomes progressively dry, his friends, the alligators, the fish, the insects, the reeds, begin to suffer more and more from the drought. From the pain of his friends, Emir learns the risk of trying to force his will upon nature. Later in this allegorical journey, he learns the same as he tries to force the wind to blow his sails only to create a tempest. The lesson is to work with nature, rather than to impose the will of thought upon it. Beliefs, then, are shorthand methods of expressing biobehavioral patterns.

Women who are involved with certain kinds of meditation that teach separation from the body to the extent of divorcing oneself from the body sometimes have trouble with birth. Birth usually requires just the opposite. It is a kind of body spirituality, a spirituality of the physical world. The journey of birth for women who have a pattern of avoiding contact with their body and of obsessing or being very intellectual may have roadblocks that need to be eliminated. This can be facilitated by relaxation training, visualization, working with guided imagery, biofeedback, applied kinesiology, acupuncture, and other techniques. They may need help making contact with their body during labor, often the dilation may stop, too, and the body process (labor) just doesn't work. These women often also have longer labors when they do deliver without intervention. The midwife may need to spend considerable time during labor working with the woman to keep contact, to keep her from "spacing out," and to keep her sentience from wandering somewhere from the process of birth.

Fear and Anxiety

Many women experience increased anxieties and fears as pregnancy nears completion.[11] Anxiety is a psychophysiological event. So is fear. Fear can decrease uterine blood flow.[12] On a long term basis, the effects of this can be lowering of fetal reserve.[12] The result of this is that the fetus will tolerate less stress during labor.

Events that would constitute normal, healthy stress for the average fetus become distress for such a compromised baby. Thus, one would expect high levels of fear and anxiety to correlate with fetal distress. This has been found to be true.

Risk screening should aim at identifying fear and anxiety. It is not sufficient, however, to make a surface search for fear and anxiety. Paradoxically, in pregnancy, a certain amount of fear and anxiety is usual. This is common in any developmental crisis in which the endpoint is unknown. Change involves a venture into the unknown which often includes anxiety.[12] Jane Roberts has written eloquently about this in poetic form regarding the life process itself which inevitably progresses toward death.[14] Total absence of fear may be as much a warning of conflict as excessive fear.

Anxiety can be expressed in the body in the form of tension and crying. An important aspect of this is openness. If I say to a tense client whose eyes are moist: "It looks as though you've been crying," and she says, "What, huh, me!" then she may be relatively emotionally inaccessible. The psychophysiological pattern related to anxiety that is most conducive to birth is a very expressive one. This is why doctors and psychologists can be fooled about the relation of anxiety to birth complications. The woman with very thick character armor who walls in her fear and anxiety may have an established biobehavioral pattern that will also appear in labor with a cervix that won't open. Such a possibility takes the form of a clinical hypotheses which then must be confirmed or denied based upon the client's past history and current status. If, in the past, the pattern is such that when the woman has high levels of fear and anxiety that she walls off inside her, physical symptoms develop (asthma, hypertension, vaginitis), this could occur during labor. Then it is important to determine if her life circumstances, beliefs, and attitudes are currently the same as that earlier time. If there has been a radical attitude change, then past history is much less reliable. Also, the presence of symptoms does not necessarily mean these symptoms would be expressed in the pelvis during labor. This must be balanced by an assessment of all the other factors.

Extreme anxiety can interfere with labor, delivery, and the care of the child. Extreme anxiety can be expressed or repressed. Such anxiety can be related to the fear of giving up a sense of unity with the child or of not having the capacity to love and care for the infant. Some women become very anxious about what sex the child will be. This can be because of pressure in the family system to have one or the other sex. Also because of women's pasts sometimes they are afraid of caring for one sex of child. One woman serves as an example of this. She was a 36 year old teacher who was having her first baby. She had had a very poor and (in her view) traumatic relationship with her mother. She did not want a girl because she felt she would "screw up" a girl child as badly as her mother did for her. She had an amniocentesis, because she wanted to abort a baby if it was a girl. When it was a girl and her husband took a strong stance against an abortion, she experienced considerable anxiety. Therapeutic work was directed toward helping her to accept the girl child and to find the source of her anxiety.

Pregnancy can be an opportunity for mastery and maturation.[4] This was very true for this patient. With prenatal therapeutic work, she had a normal labor and delivery and, not without some difficulties with postpartum, adjusted well and attached to her daughter.

Problems with Assessment for Home Birth

Couples wanting to deliver at home can present a special problem for any assessment process, especially when the consequences of making the wrong choice are so significant for everyone involved. In today's political climate, a home birth death is a very negative event. This is especially so if it could be prevented. The psychophysiological (or existential assessment process) is ideally suited for the client oriented toward personal growth and development. The decision to attend the delivery at home is one that should logically arise from the assessment process which constitutes getting to know the client. This only becomes a problem when the client demands an immediate, firm guarantee that their birth *will be* at home before the getting-acquainted process is completed and when the client takes a concrete, structural approach. This means they believe they have come to buy a home birth and it is the job of the practitioner to sell it to them. Some clients can become very manipulative in their efforts to get what they want. Sometimes this manipulation can exceed rational bounds. It is hard work to interact with such clients. There needs to be a sense of equality in the relationship. Both practitioner(s) and client(s) need to feel respected by each other. Modern society makes this difficult with its many projections about doctors and nurses. Many capable individuals discontinue their involvement with home birth because of the energy drain in dealing with such clients. This type of client is both dependent and non-trusting. Therefore, in order to "get what she wants" as she perceives it, the woman attempts to manipulate to obtain a promise for home delivery, coming from an attitude of basic distrust of the person she perceives to have what she wants. Because she is unable to form a trusting relationship, however, she precludes her "success" as she would define it. Her basic underlying belief in such a situation is that the practitioner is in power and control of her body (a diminutive belief for normal birth, i.e., the attitude of victimization) which is compounded by her distrust, which makes her inaccessible for helping her to change this belief about her body. The manipulation also, ironically, is a cover up for passivity, in the sense that the woman is very active at getting others to help her, because she believes herself to be helpless (passive).

The client must trust the practitioner and know that he or she has their desires as a first priority if felt to be medically safe. Sometimes that means commitment to the process of working together to achieve the best birth possible without making a firm commitment as to place of birth until late in the pregnancy. The problem is that some people place their personal sense of control and power in the *place* they've decided upon for birth, rather than in themselves. The people who have firmly placed their sense of power in themselves are usually the ones for whom assessment indicates high probability of a normal delivery from even early in the pregnancy. Another problem that can arise is the client confusing the practitioner's suggestion for psychophysiological psychotherapy (which can be made very diplomatically and can be called non-threatening things such as relaxation training or visualization) as indicating a contract that if they go for two sessions they can have a home birth.

We have decided that the best way to approach this difficult issue is to be sure that the therapist and the practitioner are separate in the client's perception. Thus, the therapy should not have any direct ramifications as to place of birth. The therapist's job is to do the utmost to optimize the client's chances for a normal delivery. The therapist consults the birth practitioner, but the relationship between therapist and practitioner is kept separate. We attempted to combine those functions for some of the people at Berkeley Family Health Center with less ease that we would have imagined. It works very well for the well-integrated client who will most likely have a normal delivery anyway. The problem exists for the marginally integrated client for whom assessment has indicated that her life patterns are such that there is a likelihood that the delivery may not be normal. Humans, unlike other animals, seem to have much more conscious control (often unbeknownst to them) over their physiology. Thoughts, emotions, and beliefs have physiological consequences. The body seems to work best when it is in a state of natural harmony or natural grace with the mind. Both flow in a synchronized pattern together. This makes understanding human reproduction more complex and difficult than understanding that of other mammals. Nevertheless it presents a great challenge for the expansion of consciousness for pregnant women, practitioners, and the species.

Home birth screening is easier if there are good hospital alternatives: for example, if there can be as many people (family, friends, relatives) as the parents desire, the parents are free to behave as they please, and the woman can be in any position with a comfortable double bed. It helps also if the nurses are very involved in the alternative birth concept and with the labor. When the hospital alternative is positive, it is much easier to stop worrying about place of birth and focus on preparing for the process of birth.

If home vs. hospital becomes too much the issue a kind of performance anxiety can result and become problematic, especially if the woman is relatively competitive and other friends have had home births. This is similar to the competitive phenomenon that Arthur Colman[15] describes in a group for first mothers. He reported that when some of the mothers-to-be in the group delivered and returned to the group with their babies, some of the women still pregnant became very competitive with the new mothers.

For some women the anxiety of competition may be the first in a series of steps that ultimately leads to defeat. These women usually have a history of competitive lives in which they do not see themselves as succeeding in their definition of "success." Childbirth becomes yet another failure. Beginning at home, for these women, may be exactly the wrong place. If they begin in the alternative birth center and have to go to the labor and delivery ward for a simple problem, this seems like less of a failure and is less traumatic than a transport from home to hospital. In a good alternative birth center, if the woman has a simple problem such as uterine inertia which resolves, she should be able to return to the birth center. If she had to be transported in from home, she could not return home nearly as readily.

One ethical dilemma that arises in any assessment process is when the client(s) refuse to accept the advice of the practitioner. This is especially true in the home birth arena. If a group decides to refuse to attend a delivery at home and the clients decide to do the delivery at home by themselves[6] unattended, that could, of course, lead to serious complications. The indirect effect of this can serve as a manipulation to force the practitioner into attending their delivery at home. A case example illustrates the problems inherent in this. A couple came to a midwife and asked her assistance. They told her they wouldn't go to the hospital, regardless. They would not permit her to do anything during their birth—no exams or listening to the fetal heart rate. She went to their birth anyway because she thought her presence was better than no one being there. The baby was stillborn. The district attorney attempted to prosecute the midwife, not the parents. This was associated with considerable stress for her for some time. It is possible that had she refused to go, the parents would not have relied on the myth of her presence being protective. They might have thought more about their decision. If she had not gone, things might have been the same, but then local obstetricians would have had more difficulty blaming the midwife for this mishap.

Consultation to Practitioners

One of the services the therapist can provide to the practitioner as a part of the assessment process is advice and consultation regarding how to approach clients with potentially delicate material. One approach we tried which was less successful than we had hoped was to include the therapist as an integral member of the clinical team in the client's perception. We learned from this that it is better for the therapist/assessor to not directly participate in decision-making regarding place of delivery. Rather, the therapist offers consultation with recommendations to the practitioner who must then make the final decision. Thus, the client is less able to manipulate the therapist or practitioner. The therapist is also in a more effective position to observe and comment on the practitioner's decision making process. It is usually fairly obvious when the practitioner is behaving in order to "save" the client or rescue (in Claude Steiner's sense of the rescue triangle) the client.

Some practitioners feel they don't have the right to say "no." They can't bring themselves to tell the client they haven't made a good connection. They may feel obligated to provide a good birth experience for the couple since there are few alternatives without thought to their own risk. There are people who are very litigenous who nevertheless request the practitioner to stick his or her neck out for them. These people may have to be assessed by the traditional obstetrical textbook if the practitioner is to avoid litigation. Such people tend to have the common belief that someone else is responsible for them. They tend not to take personal responsibility, but to give it to the practitioner. Then if things are not perfect, it is by definition the practitioner's fault. In alternative birth circles, the existence of such people is often denied, sometimes to the practitioner's detriment.

Importance of the Birth Counsellor

The birth counsellor is an integral and necessary member of the obstetrical team. The status of the birth counsellor is somewhat different by nature of his/her non-involvement in clinical practice.

Clients will often talk more openly about delicate issues to someone who isn't a birth attendant, who is not going to be at the birth. The birth counsellor also has the needs of the referral practice at heart, since they are her clients as well as the client. There is a symbiosis in that, if the birth attendants have a good experience, usually the client will also, and *vice versa*. The birth counsellor can often operate from a more objective framework than the practitioner. In late pregnancy when things are changing rapidly the assistance of the birth counsellor can be essential. The birth counsellor needs training in psychotherapeutic skills and needs to be able to comment on the process of care between provider and patient. He or she can say, "Hey, I see you trying to rescue her. Maybe that's going to happen in her labor. Maybe she and you will create a situation in which you'll have to rescue her." This happens.

Previous Psychiatric Treatment

A history of previous psychiatric treatment of hospitalization is often listed as a risk factor to which the practitioner should attend.[4] This is simplistic. There are patients with severe emotional problems whose bodies function very normally for them. Some clients seek psychotherapy early as a preventive measure to help them through stressful situations. Often clients who are most at risk for physical complications of delivery are those who attach a strong stigmata to psychotherapy and for whom it is very important to appear "normal." People with florid emotional disturbances often also have a belief in expressiveness and are uninhibited. This may work for their body and their labor as well.

Passivity

Women who are very passive may tend to have trouble giving birth when this is a life long pattern. If it takes the form of asking others to do or complete things for them, this may be a difficult pattern for their giving birth. The symbolic request they make to doctor or midwife is "will you please give birth for me?" Birth is a very personally active process with the woman *giving* birth, unless she is delivered (that is with forceps or C-section). Passivity is the opposite of being active, and activity is essential to the birth process. There are multiple points at which intervention can change a passive life pattern. Usually a major attitude change is required.

Self Reliance

Another important pattern is a pattern of being self-reliant as opposed to expecting other people to always help out, take charge, or take over. This is a pattern which, in many situations, the person believes they can't completely take care of the situation on their own. Self-reliance is a belief in the ability and power of the self to accomplish tasks at hand. Evidence of this belief would be a rising sense of self-identity from any challenging situation arising in a woman's life. This belief often presents a calm, confident outward appearance. It is possible to be too self-reliant. The assessment of this would consist of examining past life situations which could be successfully resolved with the help of others, but weren't because the woman was unable to ask for help. It's not necessarily problematic for birth if the woman seems to be self-reliant, lonely, and to have trouble receiving and asking for nurturing, if in the face of this attitude the woman has enough strength and belief in herself that her history is one of basic success. Sometimes the surfacing of increased needs and conflicts of pregnancy can be enough to cause such a previously successful pattern to crumble.

It is possible to accept support and help from others while

maintaining independence and self-reliance. Labor is a good time to accept others' support and help. This is not always true. Some women need to experience their own strength during labor and to be alone. Labor can bring systems, communities, couples, and families closer together, through support and help. That in itself can provoke anxiety for some women.

Sexual Beliefs

Sexual beliefs can be very important. Birth is a very sexual process. Traditional hospital settings may have developed into their often repressive nature in an effort (unconscious) to help staff manage the anxiety of this sexuality. The intimate relationships that occur and are expressed in birth can be very frightening, especially for people with obsessive, compulsive characteristics which most doctors have. People who have developed obsessive/compulsive patterns of coping with anxiety tend to "get busy" and "do things" to allay that anxiety. The anxiety of birth causes them to think of procedures they can do. The more to do, the less time there is to feel anxious and the more they can feel in control.

In the hospital, sexual anxiety is often handled by putting on gowns. Masks and hats are worn. The only person not completely covered is the woman. This allows everyone to hide from sexuality. The walls are lined with tile and kept very sterile. Women are drugged so they cannot participate in their experience. Birth is not such an intimate experience when the woman is drugged and doesn't even notice the baby's coming. Luckily, not all hospitals are this way. Some clients need to mask this sexual anxiety to give birth. Sometimes, if these women begin at home, labor stops. As soon as they get to the hospital, the baby is born. This can also be related to a fear of having a problem at home. Fear of sexuality, which can be aroused by the events of labor and birth, is hard not to acknowledge at home. In the clinical environment of the hospital that anxiety can be contained. Women who have trouble accepting their own sexuality sometimes have labors that stop at home and begin again once hospital conditions are achieved.

Single Mothers

Single mothers may need more attention as a group than their mated (married) counterparts. This could in part relate to a natural tendency to feel more ambivalent about the birth because of the anticipated stress of single parenthood. It could relate to being afraid of not having an adequate support system. Some real ambivalence about mothering may also exist. The woman may ask herself "did I make the right choice? What is it going to be like?" In general, anything that increases ambivalence about the birth process increases risk. It isn't correct to place single mothers in a high risk class by definition. It is accurate to say that, as a group, they may have more potential stress and potential ambivalence, yet each woman needs to be understood as her own person.

Couples' Conflict

Many writers, including Nadelson,[4] list couples' problems or marital or family difficulties on the list of factors for the practitioner to consider and use as a possible "red flag" to look deeper or to possibly refer the client to a therapist. Couples' problems can affect the woman physiologically in several ways. The stress of fighting with her mate may increase catecholamines and chronically decrease uterine blood flow leading to increased risk of fetal distress. In addition, we have pointed out how a desire for or a belief in a positive outcome is important to birth normally. If a relationship is "on the rocks" there is less tendency to have that. Also, there is increased ambivalence. This is especially so if the child was planned to improve an ailing relationship and this is not succeeding. It is also true if the mother is facing the unwelcome prospect (to her) of single parenthood, having begun the pregnancy expecting to be part of a two parent family. It is easy to see how such a woman, somewhere in her consciousness, could feel anger at the baby and wish it weren't there.

Family Systems Theory can help to understand the dynamics of relationships. Family Systems Theory holds that a dynamic balance exists between members of any couple, relationship, community, or socio-cultural group. This dynamic process is always in evolution. Couples are more than a simple sum of the partners. The marital see-saw is a phenomenon commonly described whereby partners pass and trade emotions. If I become hostile, my partner can become more loving. If I become loving, then she can become hostile. This means that we need to understand the relationship of the couple to properly interpret the behavior of the woman. We need to know the rules of the relationship, that is how do things work? Does the relationship require the woman to be passive and submissive in relation to her husband so that it appears she is weaker than she really is? Then we should search for what happens in a crisis. Does she allow her power to emerge or does she keep it under control in the interests of maintaining family homeostasis? The family provides a context from which individual behavior takes on more meaning. It is useful to see the woman alone and to also see her with her partner. If, for example, as in one recent case the woman did not really want a home birth but the man did and was very ego-involved in having this happen, the woman can begin to have significant performance anxiety. She really wanted to please him. This can be a set-up for potential problems. She may really want to please him but she may also be resentful that he is pushing her into birthing at home and needs a way to express this, also. If the practitioner accidently is caught in this process, there may be anxiety for the doctor or midwife as well.

Conflicts About Sexual Identity

Sexual identity is an issue everyone in our culture is forced to grapple with. It is not always easy to achieve a healthy sense of personal sexual identity. Conflicts over sexual identity can be the expression of beliefs that may also affect birth. Sexual identity issues also are bombarded during pregnancy. For most women, sexuality can remain concealed. Pregnancy "blows the cover." The fact of sexuality and sexual intercourse is apparent for everyone to see. It is impossible not to eventually notice pregnancy.

The body image changes that occur during pregnancy may also put pressure on areas that expose other beliefs that are problematic for birth. This is an issue that transcends the feminist movement in that it involves all women. The issue is one of beliefs. A woman can be very unliberated from a feminist perspective and still be very comfortable from a sexual perspective and from the standpoint of personal identity. This point was initially confusing to us. First we thought that dressing and behaving always as a sexual object (in our judgment) might be a risk. Then we realized that this was a judgment. What was important was how the woman's belief systems fit together *for her*, and what her manner of dress meant *to her*.

Another factor that contributes to ambivalence is denying the pregnancy. This may relate to a woman's feelings of herself in relation to being a woman. If pregnancy is viewed as a normal, healthy part of the sexual life cycle, it can be a very enjoyable experience. If the woman views herself as a hideous object then there can be an entirely different reaction. This obviously relates to previous acculturation. If the woman's mother always talked about or the woman experienced her mother's pregnancy and birth as dirty and humilitating, then that woman may have to work to consciously change those perceptions. The body receives in many ways these feelings of personal ambivalence or revulsion toward the body. This interferes with its natural functioning.

Nadelson[4] lists conflicts involving separation from parents as a signal area for psychological risk in pregnancy. This can also affect physiology. Midwives from Mexico have told me that the women who come with their mothers to prenatal checks are the ones who often have birth problems. This may be because they have not adequately separated from their mothers. They may have an intrinsic belief that somehow their mother will protect them from birth or from pain. Since this can't happen, their reaction to the birth may initiate a fear-panic cycle not conducive to normal birthing. Dependence is an important component of this. Such dependency usually speaks of more pervasive life patterns that are somewhat dysfunctional in terms of health. For example, one woman that BFHC turned down for home birth was planning to give birth at her mother's house even though her mother had said that wasn't acceptable to her. Her mother had said she thought birth was horrible. It was the worst thing that could happen to a woman. Everyone should be "knocked out." Yet her daughter still insisted on delivering at her mother's house. The belief in birth her mother expressed is probably existent for this woman. She may want to deliver at home exactly *because* she thinks the same as her mother and therefore wants to avoid the hospital. She may have decided the hospital is responsible for making things the way she believes them to be. She may want her mother there for support and protection against this very fearful event. The fear hormones may be so high in this situation that they will interfere with normal physiology.

Family System

If the husband is passive and fearful and doesn't want a home birth and the woman seems very strong, then that could be part of a normal physiological pattern since the woman is the one who is giving birth. Nevertheless the man may be expressing what the woman feels. She may not be able to say it, either because he's saying it for her or because she doesn't want to lose face.

Couples Issues

One couple is very interesting in relation to what we have been discussing. The husband was 55 and his wife was 24. In the relationship, he tended to play the part of "little boy" when under stress and she mothered him. His last relationship had ended after children were born and he was afraid the same would happen in this relationship. He was afraid of the baby ruining the relationship. The woman spent most of her energy during the pregnancy reassuring him. There wasn't much attention left to direct to her pregnancy. We tried to encourage them both to come together or separately for therapy, but he wouldn't come. She did, and we worked with her in terms of giving birth without him, directing more attention into delivery and focusing on herself and her baby. She needed to recognize that if he left because of the baby she couldn't ignore the baby and mother him. She had to anticipate that. When she came the baby was in breech presentation. If he would have come also, the situation would have been much more positive. As things happened, she did begin to think more about pregnancy, birth, and the baby. The baby turned vertex. Then the man withdrew severely and became very sullen. He acted angry and sarcastic toward her and the medical practitioners. In a prenatal visit he would stand at the far corner of the room and just nod his head. If he was asked to take part, he would say, "I guess not." Then the woman changed again and the man seemed to brighten. She stopped talking and thinking about the birth and the baby and began to focus her awareness predominantly on him again. Soon thereafter the baby turned back to breech. She had a Cesarean section because of a malposition of the breech that made vaginal breech delivery too risky. During that time her husband imagined that medical and hospital personnel were treating his wife and baby badly. He set himself up in a belligerent way to protect the two of them from the rest of the world.

Trust

Trust is a very positive factor that mitigates against many of the other factors we have discussed. Likewise, lack of trust is significant. If the practitioner learns the client is withholding important information or presenting things that aren't the case, then there is a clear issue of lack of trust. This is related to a risk signal frequently quoted, included by Nadelson,[4] which is, "previous poor relationships with physicians." A history of problems with physicians or litiginous behavior mitigates against the possibility of trust (even when to some extent the previous physician was largely responsible for the poor relationship). Midwives may feel exempt from this. In actuality, this is a false feeling of security. The midwife may be seen as a savior who is to rescue her from doctors. When the midwife is human rather than divine, the client may become very angry, very quickly. This is particularly true if their view has been that the problem with previous negative birth experiences was all the fault of the doctor or the hospital, and they have given the midwife responsibility for this birth being completely normal. One client desiring a home birth was attending three birthing services because she had state funding for her care (Medi-Cal) and she wanted to always take the option that seemed best, while presenting her story three separate times.

Ability to Form Good Relationship

The ability to relate well to others (spouse, practitioner, friends) seems to be important. This may be because it bespeaks of generally successful modes of coping and adapting.

Spiritual Beliefs

Spiritual beliefs can have very important impacts. If the client believes that birth is a trauma then it may be difficult for her to put the baby through a traumatic experience. I do not believe that birth is necessarily traumatic. I have seen births at which the baby's head is born and the baby opens its eyes and looks around. Then the shoulders are born and the baby doesn't cry. It is put on the mother's chest and it starts to crawl up between her breasts and be very happy. There is no trauma there.

In addition, the crying experience is also one of adaptation for the newborn, as crying opens the lungs, and clears them and other air breathing passageways of mucous. Crying is not necessarily an indication of trauma, but rather an indication of expressive and healthy adaptation to the world outside the womb. In cases in which the birth has been difficult for the baby physiologically, perhaps, traumatic robust crying is not the result, but rather lack of this healthy adaptive response is present in conjunction with a physiologically depressed looking baby.

There is one spiritual community in California that, of 40 planned home births, there were four deliveries at home and 36 hospital transports. The one overriding similarity among these women in general, and among most members of this spiritual community, was the belief that being born was a traumatic and difficult experience.

Fear

Complete absence of fear is as worrisome as total fear. There is a healthy amount of fear. One study showed that the more fearful dreams a woman had during pregnancy with her first baby the easier the labor went.[17] If somebody always wants to talk about complications, that may be a sign of a strong belief that nature is imperfect or that they will have problems. I hope I'm getting the picture across because there's a certain normal, good learning process about birth that has to take place and somewhat includes learning about what could go wrong. People who say they have no fear may not be completely aware of their own emotion. There's inevitably a kind of fear involved in birth in that the life of being single is forever ended. Upon becoming a parent the free life of not being one is forever lost. From that point on, there is total responsibility for another human being. There's the death of the old relationship between the couple. No longer can they go easily away to Lake Tahoe for the weekend. From then on the kids are in tow. Recreation is very different, also. They can't go skiing like they once did. Camping in the Sierras isn't as easy. There's a real death of the old lifestyle that has to be worked through. Birth involves the possibility of death which the parents must come to terms with in some way. Denial of fear prevents the kind of working through and yielding that allows birth to happen readily. Without the yielding the natural balance of yin and yang or of archetypal masculine and feminine is no longer present—a balance so necessary to the androgyny of the process. Death must be faced in the possibilities of birth. To deny its possibility may create the show of absence of fear, while to continually fear its possibility may create excessive fear. Facing both doors of life is intrinsic in the birth process. To face the possibility of death may be fearful, but can be worked through to a basic acceptance of what life does have to offer us. The same is true of fear of abnormalities. They can and generally are worked through by the majority of women experiencing normal childbirth, as something that is unlikely, yet a possibility, over which they may have little control. The resolution to this dilemma of facing death, yet not fearing it or necessarily expecting it, is the phenomenon of yielding to the unknown in a trusting manner. It is a basic attitude of trust in the universe. A healthy or normal fear of the unknown can yield to trust in the universe.

Change

Sometimes clients cannot accept help easily. They may become very angry at their practitioner for suggesting they need extra help and aren't already perfect. They may leave the first practitioner in anger and upset. Nevertheless, they can accept the suggestions to begin the change and, by the time they arrive at the office of the second practitioner, have already begun that change process. They are not the same person who left Jill's office for Jack. Jack could think Jill was crazy for ever thinking wrong of Jane, who has a wonderful birth with Jack. When Jill hears of Jane's success, Jill could think she was all wrong. Jill can feel much better if she realizes that Jill helped Jane begin a process that Jack could help her complete. Jill can feel happy that she could do this service for Jane, even though Jane may have a "see, I showed you, didn't I?" attitude toward Jill. In fact, this very attitude of needing to show Jill may have given Jane sufficient motivation to carry through what she needed to do to have a normal birth. This is because sometimes clients begin with one practitioner and are very dependent upon that person. There is a limit to how far they can grow because of excessive dependence. However, the dependence may have been necessary for the initial learning period. If the first practitioner will not help with the birth at home, that fact can help the client become angry and take their own power back, to break the dependence which they initially needed. The practitioner may not have ever wanted it in the first place. Then the client can take her power and find someone new who will help her because she is a new person. She has changed. She has worked through her dependency need, and is ready to be self-reliant.

Screening for risk, then, is not to take the form of hard and fast prediction, without taking into account the potential for change. In cases where assessment has revealed the need for change to avoid potential risk in childbirth, the practitioner can view him or herself as a possible change agent. As a change agent, the practitioner may be able to open new vistas to the client, by facilitating her own deepest resources. This facilitation may take the form of emotional support, confrontation, demystification, referral for relaxation/visualization therapy, psychotherapy, and/or effective childbirth classes. Whatever the form, the acknowledgement of birth as a learning experience deepens a woman's resources for learning more about herself, facilitating her own personal growth into motherhood, and beyond. This is what this book is about.

REFERENCES

1. Bibring, G. Some Considerations of the Psychological Processes in Pregnancy. *Psychoanalytic Study of the Child* 14: 113, 1959.

2. Erikson, E. *Childhood and Society*. New York, W. W. Norton, 1950.

3. Bibring, G., Dwyer, T., Huntington, D., et all. A Study of the Earliest Mother-Child Relationship, *Psychoanalytic Study of the Child* 16:9, 1961.

4. Nadelson, C. "Normal" and "Special" Aspects of Pregnancy, *Obstet. Gynecol.* 41 (4):611-620, 1973.

5. Deutsch, H. *The Psychology of Women, Motherhood*. Vol. 2 New York, Grune & Stratton, 1945.

6. Pleshette, N., Asch, S., and Chase, J. A Study of Anxieties During Pregnancy, Labor and Early and Late Perpeurium. *Bull. New York Academy of Medicine* 32:436, 1956.

7. Bibring, G., Dwyer, T., Huntington, D., et al. A Study of the Earliest Mother-Child Relationship, *Psychoanalytic Study of the Child* 16:9, 1961.

8. Daniels, P. S. and Lessow, H. Severe Postpartum Reactions: An Interpersonal View. *Psychosomatics* 5:21, 1964.

9. Caplan, G. Psychological Aspects of Maternity Care. *Am. J. Public Health* 47:25, 1957.

10. Boss, M. *Existential Foundations of Medicine and Psychology*. New York: Aronson, 1978.

11. Benedek, T. Sexual Function in Women, Chap. 37, *American Handbook of Psychiatry*, Vol. I. New York, Basic Books.

12. Mehl, L. E. Psychophysiological Aspects of Pregnancy, Chap. 3. Feher, L., *The Psychology of Birth*. London, Souvenir, 1980.

13. Mehl, L. E. and Peterson, G. Existential Risk Screening. P. Ahmed, ed. *Psychosocial Aspects of Pregnancy*. New York, Elsevier—North Holland, 1981.

14. Roberts, J. *Dialogues of the Mortal Self in Time*. Englewood Cliffs, Prentice-Hall, 1977.

15. Colman, A. D. Psychology of a First-Baby Group, *Int. J. Group Psychotherapy* 74-83, Jan. 21, 1971.

16. Roberts, J. *Emir's Education in the Proper Use of Magical Powers*. New York, Delacorte Press/Eleanor Friede, 1979.

17. For more information on dream research in pregnancy, see Lismay, J., *Dreams and Pregnancy*, Doctoral Dissertation, California School of Professional Psychology, Berkeley, 1980.

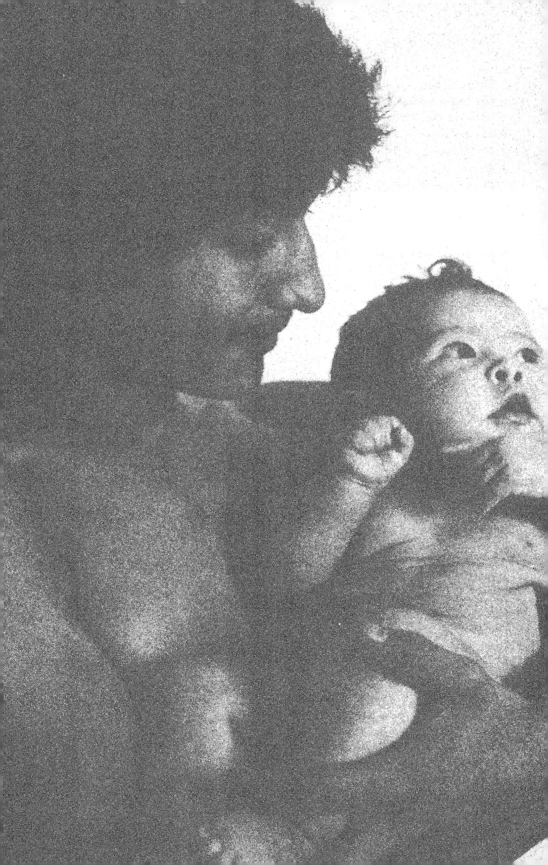

Chapter Thirteen

Results of Prospective Holistic Prenatal Risk Screening

Lewis Mehl, MD, Ph.D
Jo McRae, Ph.D
Laura Grimes. MA, MD
Gayle Peterson, MSSW, LCSW

Carl Simonton and his colleagues [1] state:

"We all participate in our own health through our beliefs, our feelings, and our attitudes toward life, as well as in more direct ways, such as through exercise and diet. In addition, our response to medical treatment is influenced by our beliefs about the effectiveness of the treatment and by the confidence we have in the medical team."

The Simontons arrived at that stance through their own work with cancer patients at the Cancer Counselling and Research Center in Fort Worth, Texas. Separately, through our work in Madison, Wisconsin and in the San Francisco Bay Area (now at the Holistic Psychotherapy and Medical Group) we had been arriving at much the same conclusion for the childbirth process. In childbirth, health means a normal, happy delivery. Our beliefs about ourselves, our bodies, the world, and the birth process influence the physical outcome of birth. This includes our beliefs in the medical team chosen to attend us.

The Simontons found that if cancer patients could mobilize their own resources and actively participate in their recovery, they could well exceed their life expectancy and significantly alter the quality of life. Our clinical experience was the same for obstetrical patients. If women who would not be expected to have a normal birth could be helped to mobilize their resources and to actively participate in preparing emotionally and physically for their delivery, they could well exceed the expectations of their obstetrician.

Carl Simonton came upon his conclusions during his residency at the University of Oregon Medical School. He noticed that some cancer patients who said they wanted to live would act as if they did not. This was our observation as well. Women who were at risk for premature labor would ignore the advice of their physician and continue to be active and avoid bed rest. Women who were becoming hypertensive would ignore the advice of their doctor to cut back and would continue to work at high pressure jobs for long hours until their condition had deteriorated to an extreme level.

Simonton also noticed cancer patients whose medical prognosis indicated that, with treatment, they could look forward to many more years of life, "Yet, while they affirmed again and again that they had countless reasons to live, these patients showed greater apathy, depression, and attitude of giving up than did a number of others diagnosed with terminal disease." This was more subtle with obstetrical patients, since their "condition" was less severe. Nevertheless, a number of patients asserted themselves who had every reason medically to have a normal birth, yet they did not. The traditional medical explanation was of a random wastage that nature interposed upon the reproductive process. This is the same explanation traditional medical wisdom gives for why certain patients develop cancer. "Random unluckiness," one doctor remarked to me. This did not fit our observations. As we looked deeper, we observed that despite the best physical conditions for birth, a variety of attitudes and beliefs appeared which were shared among these patients. These included beliefs that their body would fail them, previous biobehavioral patterns that resulted in physical disease, and a variety of other conflicts. Our search for these proceeded, in wrong direction, until we began to realize that the birth outcome made total sense when viewed in the context of an overall gestalt of the woman's life. Initially, the psychological approach to identifying risk factors had been helpful and useful, but was not as accurate as this new approach. Nevertheless, an approach that included both was necessary to train others regarding what specifics to look for to achieve that gestaltist overview. A common problem, however, was that some of the practitioners we attempted to train could not make the transition from a psychological trait view to an overall gestalt view.

High Risk Screening

The identification of high risk pregnancies to anticipate labor complications is a major thrust of current obstetrical research. Aubrey and Pennington[2] state that "the common goal of modern obstetrics and pediatrics is to maximize the quality of fetal, newborn, and infant life in such a manner as to give every individual conceived the greatest opportunity for optimal physical, mental, and emotional development." Problems arise in planning the appropriate allocation of health care manpower, technology, and financial resources. Good high risk screening can allow for better use of limited resources for the optimum good of pregnant women and their babies.

Several attempts have been made at recognition and grading of high-risk pregnancies.[3-5] The fetuses of mothers with a history of high-risk pregnancy tend to be more acidotic than those whose mothers had a normal course during pregnancy.[6] Statistically significant differences for both one and five-minute Apgar scores ($p < 0.000005$) were found when low risk (Goodwin score ≤ 3) were compared with high risk (Goodwin score ≤ 6) women.[7] Goodwin's score ranges from 0 to 10 with the higher risk receiving the higher score. The score is the sum of three major components: previous obstetric history, ranged from 0 to 3; present obstetric history, ranged from 0 to 3; and gestational age, ranged from 0 to 4. Further divisions of the Goodwin's score did not reveal any significant differences. A correlation coefficient was found between the high-risk score and the one-minute Apgar score of -0.3718 ($p < 0.001$), and between the high-risk score and the five minute Apgar score of -0.2668 ($p < 0.001$). Similar correlations were found between high risk score and umbilical artery blood pH at birth, significant at the $p = 0.01$ level. Yeh[7] found that with a Goodwin score of 3 or less (which indicated low risk), 45% of depressed babies (Apgar 7 at 1 minute) were predicted properly and 75% of non-depressed babies were predicted properly. At 5 minutes, the correct prediction of depressed babies was 60% and of non-depressed babies, 75%. Using the score of 4 or more as an indicator of high risk, throughout labor fetal scalp pH was significantly different between the two groups and there was a significantly higher occurrence of late deceleration patterns in the "high-risk" group ($p = 0.001$ by t test), but no statistical difference in the occurrence of normal and variable deceleration patterns.

Butler and Alderman[8] and Shapiro, et al.[9] report that the major factors affecting perinatal mortality and morbidity are age, race, marital status, parity, past obstetric performance, medical-obstetric ills, reproductive tract abnormalities, nutrition, psychological state, and socioeconomic status.

Aubrey and Pennington[2] describe the use of Nesbitt's Maternal and Child Health Care (MCHC) Index based upon the above factors. When corrected for congenital anomalies, more that 50% of all perinatal mortality and morbidity arises from the 29% of the clinic population found to be at risk by the Index. Over 50% of all maternal complications and 60% of all primary Cesarean sections arose from the same high risk group. When a Labor Index was added and one year's perinatal deaths analyzed and corrected for anomalies, 52% of the perinatal deaths would have been identified by the Labor Index. Aubrey and Pennington state that 20-30% of problem newborns originate from low risk populations.

Aubrey and Pennington's experience was that past obstetric history, medical-obstetric disorders, pelvic or generative tract disorders, and socioeconomic factors were the most significant predictors.[2] Maternal age, race, marital status, parity and nutrition were fairly good, but emotional and psychological factors were definitely not worth consideration. Our data and experience presented in this paper suggests very different conclusions. The possible reasons for such discrepancies will be discussed.

Rantakallio[10] administered a questionnaire to 12,000 mothers during pregnancy in North Finland in 1966. It reviewed biological characteristics, past obstetric history and socioeconomic factors. Fourteen percent of the obstetric population could be identified in which the fetal growth rate was slower, birth weights smaller, and the risk of low-birth weight infancy more than 2½ times higher than the remainder of the population.

Methods

The methods used in this study are somewhat unusual and will be described in detail. We favor the use of a phenomenological methodology and its practical application in grounded theory.[11-14] We are actually measuring the success rate of our group of practitioners using semi-objective guidelines in predicting the risk status of a group of women who are medically at low-risk. Through this we are indirectly measuring the role of psychosocial variables in contributing to obstetrical risk.

This approach is, at the onset, very different from the modern obstetrical practice which generated the data discussed in the high risk section. Each woman is considered individually as her own case study. She is not just an obstetrical patient with assumptions already having been made regarding her similarity to all other members of the class "obstetrical patients." She is a total human being who must be understood as such and within the context of other human beings with whom she has developed and maintains intimate relationships. She cannot be compared to a mass of other such individuals and scored on various factors in comparison to that mass, such as is common in modern obstetrics. This is similar to what the Simontons describe as happening for "cancer patients."

We have called our approach psychophysiological since it includes factors related to beliefs, emotions, behavior and physiology. We observed that many experienced clinicians had an intuitive sense of which women might have problems during labor. In some instances, they could accurately predict *which* complication would occur without any *seeming* objective basis for such predication. Aubrey and Pennington[2] state that "every experienced clinician comes to a point of clinical judgement which he exercises depending upon his own evaluation of the patient's circumstances." Many agree this requires a certain intuitive ability. In previous research on home birth[15,16] it was apparent that there were anecdotal reports of women who had been screened out of home birth by the practitioners on non-objective grounds (intuitive) who then developed severe complications during labor in the hospital. It seemed logical to believe there could be *other* variables which clinicians can recognize and respond to, even though not necessarily *consciously*. We interviewed clinicians who had engaged in such successful predictions and questioned them closely regarding the details of those experiences. We reviewed our own cumulative experience of 500 deliveries from 1973–1977 and examined the case histories of all those women who had begun labor at home and required hospital transport. Some very detailed observational data came from a study of the effects of the birth experience on parental attachment[17,18]. Emphasis was placed on every aspect of the woman's life, including:

1. Past medical history
2. Emotional life history
3. Predominant behavioral patterns
4. Biobehavioral patterns (discovered by matching the emotional behavioral history on one piece of paper to the body (medical) history on a parallel piece of paper)
5. Coping styles
6. Family medical history
7. Nutrition
8. Stress
9. Energy in relation to strength and yielding
10. Discongruity among personal belief systems
11. Biogenetic contribution and other factors

Interaction among content variables was stressed, and an attempt was made to discover underlying processes that can be viewed as common themes throughout life.

To understand our methodology, the reader is referred to *Holistic Prenatal Care, Mind and Matter,* and to the workshops offered through Psychophysiological Associates to teach this model. In particular, the Holistic Prenatal Care and Risk Screening workshop and the Practical Holism during Pregnancy and Birth would be very helpful.

Figure 1 illustrates our view more clearly and shows the final predictive scale we use in the study.[21] The fulcrum seems to be an ideal model to illustrate our approach. The weights on the left side of the balance represent those risk factors the woman brings into the pregnancy. The fulcrum begins at a certain place on the balance. By working with a client, we can change the position of the fulcrum and potentially balance some of the risk factors she brings into the pregnancy. As the fulcrum concept illustrates, the client can augment or reduce the risk factors she brings to the pregnancy through her lifestyle, behavior, and affective set. The numbers on the right of the figure represent predictions. These are general rather than specific predictions.

Figure 1

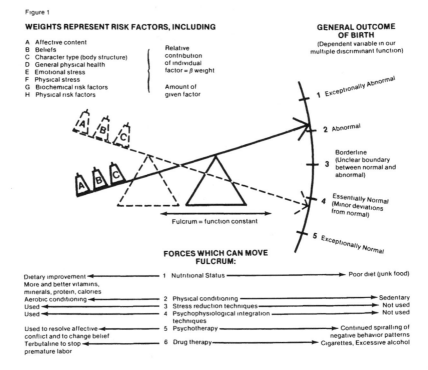

Figure 2 further illustrates the model upon which our predictions are based.[21] A set of general factors shown to the left of the figure create an energized state which is then capable of producing a specific complication (the right of the figure) based upon specific conditions present in the organism and the environment. This general-to-specific outcome model seems to be an attribute of creative systems. It has been well studied in the chemical thermodynamic literature and has been utilized in chemical systems. A given set of general conditions sets the stage for a chemical reaction to occur and results in an energized molecule at a high level of potential. At this phase of the reaction there are highly unstable intermediates which may be identified only with some diffiuclty. Then a set of stable compounds arises from the intermediate. Catalysts in organic chemistry correspond to our fulcrum in the psychophysiological approach to risk-factor screening.

Figure 2

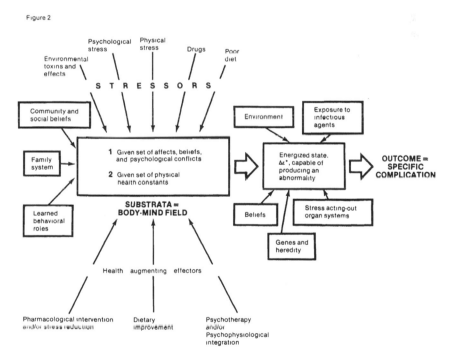

Our original interest was in improving the ability of practitioners at BFHC to predict in advance which women could safely deliver at home and which should deliver within a hospital. The development of hospital Alternative Birth Centers (ABC)

allowed an environment in which hospital deliveries could be approached in the same style as home deliveries. The main difference was that the mother was not in her own home. Prior to this, one had to choose between a good emotional experience at home or a sometimes safer experience in the hospital, but a significant emotional risk. With the development of the ABC, screening could be done more effectively, since there was a very positive alternative to offer women who were not medically high risk, but who still might develop, based upon other considerations, a complication during labor that might require hospital intervention.

This approach arises naturally from a philosophy that birth complications are not a purely physical problem, but rather a problem of the total person, including mind, body, beliefs, emotions, and environment. Beliefs, emotions, and attitudes play a significant role both in *susceptibility* to birthing problems and in changing or eliminating factors that predispose to such problems. Birth problems are often an indication of problems elsewhere in the person's life.

Simonton states that "If the total integrated system of mind, body, and emotions, which constitutes the whole person, is not working in the direction of health, then purely physical interventions may not succeed." This is as true for obstetrics as for oncology. Effective programs for any medical specialty must focus on the total person and not just the disease or condition.

Expectancy in obstetrics, either positive or negative, can play a very significant role in determining outcome. It may be possible that with early identification of risk and treatment aimed at minimizing these risks, birth complications can be prevented much more than at present. Doctors often condition patients to expect certain outcomes (such as forceps or Cesarean section) through the doctor continually telling the woman she may need such intervention. Or, if the woman spontaneously mentions wanting a normal, happy birth, he/she reminds her of all the things that can go wrong and tries to make sure she doesn't expect a normal birth, so that if "things do go wrong" she won't be disappointed. The same approach is used for natural childbirth. The doctor reminds the woman often that she doesn't have to succeed and that many don't so that she won't be disappointed or feel guilty for using drugs when, inside herself, she knew she could have birthed without drugs. The holistic approach differs in that we are always working toward the best possible outcome while acknowledging other possibilities. In assessing a woman as potentially benefiting from holistic intervention, we are not judging her or "programming" her toward a complication. Every effort is aimed at movement toward health.

Modern medicine may be creating a biology of hopelessness. Simonton, et al[1] describe this same approach for cancer patients. They state, "A negative expectation will prevent the possibility of disappointment, but it may also contribute to a negative outcome that was not inevitable . . . Without hope the person has only hopelessness (a feeling that . . . is already too much a part of the cancer patient's life and personality). This contributes to the sense of helplessness."

Table III

Medical Risk Factors
Not Present in This Population

High Risk Prenatal Factors

I. CARDIOVASCULAR AND RENAL

Toxemia
Hypertension
Renal disease
Heart disease

II. METABOLIC

Diabetes
Previous endocrine ablation
Thyroid disease, uncontrolled

III. PREVIOUS HISTORIES

Previous fetal exchange transfusion for Rh
Previous cesarean section

IV. ANATOMIC ABNORMALITIES

Uterine malformation
Incomplete cervix
Abnormal fetal position
Polyhydramnios

V. MISCELLANEOUS

Multiple pregnancy
Sickle cell disease
Rh sensitization only
Positive serology
Severe anemia (9 gm. Hgb)
Excessive use of drugs
Pulmonary disease, moderate to severe
Alcohol (moderate)
Active bacterial infection
Non-reactive non-stress test
Positive Oxytocin Challenge Test

Population

All women were medically low risk. None of the factors listed in Table III were present. The women included in this study were receiving care from a low fee community clinic in Berkeley, California (written about elsewhere 19). These women were 65% publically funded (Medi-Cal) and 35% privately funded. The racial mixture was predominantly Caucasian, with 20% racial minorities. Comprehensive family health care services were provided in conjunction with prenatal and birthing services. Clients included are those delivering between July, 1977 and April, 1980, when changes in state funding forced the clinic to close.

Table IV

Prediction Groups

5 — Entirely normal delivery expected without the need for any medical or psychological intervention. Could be at home.

4 — Probably normal delivery, but with possible/probable need for psychological intervention which would most likely be effective and/or minor medical intervention (episiotomy, etc.).

3 — Unpredictable, or expect complication which could be probably handled at home, but we would prefer not to. Would much prefer hospital ABC and will do what we can to accomplish that.

2 — Expect complicated delivery with need for hospital intervention. Would not do at home.

1 — Expect major complication in which every second is of the essence.

Table IV restates the prediction categories.[21] The final prediction score is developed at 36 weeks by group consensus based upon the criteria previously listed.

Ratings

Outcomes at labor and delivery were assigned to the same categories as predictions, on the basis of objective data abstracted by blind raters from each patient's chart, according to the severity, not number, of complications.

Data Analysis

Frequency of cases in each category and X^2 analysis of predicted versus actual outcomes were then performed. The SPSS system of programs was used as available on the University of California, Berkeley, CDC 6400 computer system.

A general prediction was made that a pregnant woman could have a complication of four gradations of severity. This was predicted on the belief that a variety of general and specific factors render a woman susceptible to having a problem. A specific complication then arises based on specific conditions present in the organism and the environment. In other words, we predicted that the individual's general threshold for susceptability will be surpassed by the added stress of labor or during labor. This model is discussed more fully in *Holistic Prenatal Care.*

This approach arose naturally from a philosophy that birth complications were not merely random, physical phenomena, but an expression of the total person, including mind, body, beliefs, emotions, and environment. Beliefs, emotions, and attitudes were thought to play a significant role both in susceptibility to birthing problems and in changing or eliminating factors that might predispose to such problems.

For the purpose of simplifying our data, each client was assigned to a prediction category once each trimester. That category to which they were assigned at the 36th week of pregnancy was used for this research as the predicted risk category. Table 1 reproduces the categories of prediction. Assignments were made by group consensus of the researchers based on data obtained from routine prenatal exams, childbirth classes, and special research interview, as well as information provided by clinicians. In general, before a factor was considered significant for an individual woman, it should have occurred before in her past with negative physiological consequences.

Results

Table V

200 Prenatal Prospective Predictions Made

			Group
Predicted entirely normal birth	32	(16%)	5
Predicted probably normal or minor problems which could be handled at home	54	(27%)	4
Equal probability of normal vs. abnormal, or problems expected which we would definitely not want at home.	48	(24%)	3
Predicted complications requiring hospital intervention	66	(33%)	2
Predicted serious complication obviating transport time.	0	(0%)	1

Table V illustrates the distribution of the first 200 predictions made. Table VI shows the results of group 5 predictions. All patients predicted to have a completely normal delivery did so. Table VII shows the actual results for prediction group.[4] The cumulative total percentage of women predicted to have reasonably normal deliveries (who could theoretically deliver at home) was 96%. The two exceptions had complications which were not of an immediately urgent nature.

Table VI

Results of Prediction Group 5

Predicted entirely normal birth	32	
Had entirely normal birth	32	(100%)

Figure 3 **OUTCOMES OF PREDICTION GROUP 5**
(predicted entirely normal delivery)

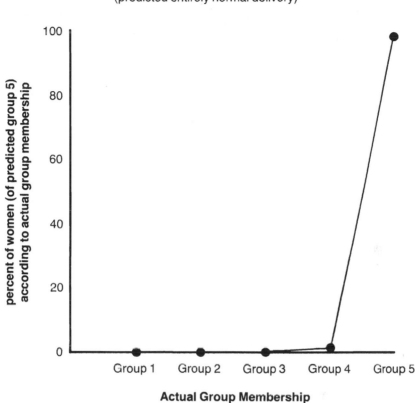

Actual Group Membership

Table VII

Results of Prediction Group 4

Number in Prediction Group 4	54	(27%)
Percent who had entirely normal births		31%
Percent who were in actual group 4		65%
Percent in actual Group 3		2%
Percent in actual Group 2		2%
Successful prediction for alternative style delivery (predicted Group 4 or 5 remains 4 or 5)		95%

Figure 4   **OUTCOMES OF PREDICTION GROUP 4**
(predicted minor medical or psychological intervention)

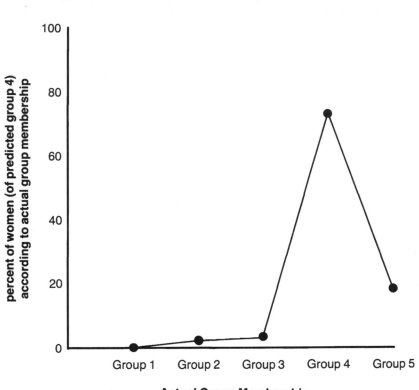

Table VIII shows the actual outcome of prediction Group 3. This group had the greatest variance which one would expect, since those clients who were enigmas to our prediction system were placed in this group. The distribution was virtually a normal one. Nevertheless, if a score of 3 was used as indicating inadvisability of home delivery, women obtaining this score could do well at home approximately 39% of the time and 61% of the time would do best inside hospital facilities. Combining Prediction Groups 1, 2, and 3 shows the total false positive rate was 24% and false negative rate was 4%. The false positive rate may be artificially high since some of these women who did well in the hospital alternative birth center may have needed the extra support and structure provided there to feel comfortable enough to allow delivery to occur without inertia. The results thus indicate that 76% of the women who would have been cleared for home delivery on medical grounds and who were judged at risk on psychophysiological grounds, did in fact need the hospital. Fifty-seven percent of the medically low-risk women became high-risk during labor. This compares to 4% in a sample of women we studied in Wisconsin. From these results we would hypothesize that other factors are clearly important in defining the low risk pregnancy than those commonly recognized.

Figure 5   **OUTCOMES OF PREDICTION GROUP 3**
(predicted portable technology or equi-potential prediction*)

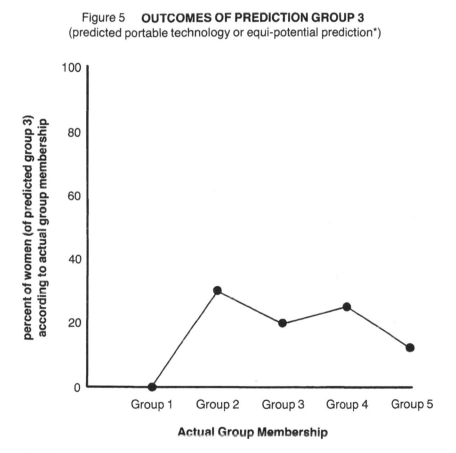

*equi-potential prediction implies that our prediction was that the woman could probably equally move either toward normalcy or complication

Table VIII

Results of Prediction Group 3

Number of women in Prediction Group 3	48	(24%)
Percent in actual Group 5		13%
Percent in actual Group 4		26%
Percent in actual Group 3		24%
Percent in actual Group 2		34%
Percent in actual Group 1		3%

Figure 6 **OUTCOMES OF PREDICTION GROUP 2**
(predicted major hospital intervention)

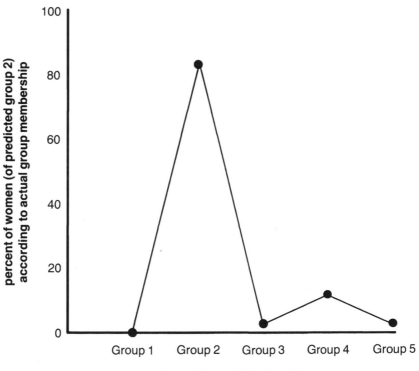

Table IX presents the result of Prediction Group 2. We can see that the success rate in predicting this group is high (85%). This group also accounts for a very high percentage of total complications, and for virtually all the serious problems.

Table IX

Results of Prediction Group 2

Number predicted to be in Group 2	66
Percent actually in Group 5	4%
Percent actually in Group 4	9%
Percent actually in Group 3	0%
Percent actually in Group 2	85%
Percent actually in Group 1	2%

Tables X and XI show the prediction groups and the actual results for the larger sample of 315 women. Figures 3 through 6 graphically diagram the results for each prediction group. No patients were predicted to have life-threatening complications; three women did. All three of these women came from prediction group 3. The complications consisted of a stillbirth, a very premature infant who died at 2 days of life, and an emergency Cesarean section for severe fetal distress.

One hundred fifteen women were predicted as needing hospital-level (high technology) intervention; 122 actually did — most for uterine inertia. The Cesarean section rate was 15% of the total sample and was derived soley from actual group 2. The majority of the other women in actual group 2 received oxytocin augmentation or induction.

A total of 84 women were rated either as unpredictable or as needing portable-level technology intervention. Thirty-one women actually needed portable-level technology. The remaining 53 split almost evenly between requiring high-level technology intervention or having normal or essentially normal deliveries. Seventy-seven women were predicted as having essentially normal deliveries, whereas 90 actually did. Thirty-nine women were predicted as having entirely normal deliveries; 69 actually did.

Using our rating system, 36.5% of the women were predicted

as being high risk for labor; 39.7% were actually high risk. Only two patients rated as 4 or higher actually became 2 or lower in their actual outcome — both requiring uncomplicated oxytocin induction for prolonged rupture of membranes. All medically low-risk patients did begin their labor in the hospital-alternative birth room. The results are skewed toward the false-positive direction. Only 36.8% were predicted in the two "normal" ranges; 50.4% actually were. Ninety percent of those women predicted as requiring high-level technology actually did require such intervention.

Table X
PREDICTED CATEGORIES

		Predicted		Actual	
Category label	**Code**	**Absolute**	**Frequency**	**Absolute**	**Frequency**
Life threatening complication in which time is of the essence	1	0	0.0	3	1.0%
Major complication requiring hospital technology	2	115	36.5%	122	39.7%
Unpredictable or portable technology complication best handled in hospital	3	84	26.6%	31	9.8%
Minor intervention easily handled out of hospital	4	77	24.4%	90	28.6%
Completely normal delivery	5	39	12.4%	69	21.9%
		315	100%	315	100%

Using our criteria of a predictive rating of 4 or more as a criterion for out-of-hospital birth, there would have been a 1.06% hospital transfer rate. This represented one woman transported for prolonged rupture of membranes without labor. This woman had a normal delivery after oxytocin induction.

Using our criterion of 3 or lower to indicate the need for hospital delivery resulted in 87% correct prediction of a delivery requiring intervention that can only be done in the hospital. Those classified as "unpredictable" were screened into the hospital, and, in fact, two of the three life-threatening complications emerged from this group. These included two fatal cord injuries to infants.

Traditional medical screening would have been correct 36.9% of the time among this group of women in predicting normalcy. We were right 95.5% of the time. Traditional screening would have correctly picked none of the 90 complications we correctly identified.

Table XI
RESULTS

Count Row pct Col pct Tot pct	Actual Outcome					
	Life-threatening complication	Major complication requiring hospitalization	Unpredictable or best served in hospital	Minor intervention	Normal	Row total
Predicted life-threatening complications	0 0 0 0	0 0 0 0	0 0 0 0	0 0 0 0	0 0 0	0
Complications requiring hospital management	1 0.9 33.3 0.3	96 83.5 78.7 30.5	3 2.6 10.0 1.0	11 9.6 12.2 3.5	4 3.5 5.8 1.3	115 36.5
Unpredictable	2 2.4 66.7 0.6	24 28.9 19.7 7.6	25 20.2 80.3 7.9	21 25.3 23.3 6.7	12 14.5 17.4 3.8	84 26.6
Minor intervention	0 0 0 0	2 2.6 1 6 0.6	3 3.9 10.0 1.0	57 74.0 63.3 18.1	15 19.5 21.7 4.8	77 24 4
Normal	0 0 0 0	0 0 0 0	0 0 0 0	1 2.6 1.1 .3	38 97.4 55.1 12.1	39 12.4
Column total	3 1.0	122 38.7	31 9.8	90 28.6	69 21.9	315 100.0

Discussion

The success of predicting which women among 315 low-risk women will have birth problems is validating for the model we have been describing. To most obstetricians all of these complications would have been unsuspected and would have increased, perhaps, their belief in the unpredictability of nature. This may be because of lack of time to get to know the patient. Also people may be very nice and friendly, but still have emotional factors which are not conducive to normal birthing. In terms of this, a surgeon recently remarked to me, "It's the nice women that get breast cancer." I knew his patient and some of her dynamics which helped one readily understand her disease. On the surface, she was very nice, which explains why, without deeper probing, this surgeon felt as he did. His belief also was that people who get diseases should somehow be obviously bad or nasty if psychological factors do play a part. Further examination shows that there is nothing to recommend this belief at all as holding any veracity.

The tendency in our predictions was the complete avoidance of the life-threatening complication category. Even so, only 33 subjects (10.5%) in the entire study had more complicated outcomes than those predicted for them. Two hundred and fifteen (68.3%) were predicted accurately, and 66 (21.0%) were predicted to have more complicated outcomes than those actually occurring. Thus, in our rating scheme, we were more likely to take unnecessary precautions than otherwise. Perhaps, had the "unpredictable" category been eliminated, the tendency toward caution would have been even more pronounced.

The ability to predict complications in a medically low-risk population is helpful in reducing morbidity and mortality from improper choice of delivery setting. Even in the hospital setting, morbidity can be reduced by anticipating and alleviating those factors that may become a source of stress to the woman in labor, whether through active psychotherapy, a congenial hospital setting, or appropriate medical intervention. Such measures may even have a beneficial effect on later infant-parent relations. More importantly, a holistic view provides increased opportunities for prenatal intervention to descrease risk and for maximum benefit to the individual.

The approach described here fits within what is popularly called holistic health—a complete view and treatment of the whole person in medical care. What is important is a recognition of the methodology of working from the general to the specific, rather than the usual medical approach of specific to general. In this paper we begin with a general notion of how psychosocial factors affect birth and show that this general model can be successfully applied.

From these results several important concepts emerge:

1. Psychological factors do seem to be associated with complications of labor. We conceptualize psychological factors and psychosocial factors such as the ones we have studied as a crucial part of a series of hierarchical systems with body manifestations. To understand the system whereby physical complications of birth appear, it is necessary to include psychosocial factors.

In separate studies[21] we have shown that psychotherapeutic treatment can reduce birth complications. This approach is similar to that the Simontons[1] use for cancer, in which they have reported good results.

2. Obstetrical services should have a skilled mental health professional as part of the team.

3. Time spent in developing an open, trusting relationship between health practitioner and client is both health-effective and cost-effective. This probably explains in part improved outcomes of lay midwives over physicians in some areas and also the success of various nurse-midwifery projects, particularly the Madera County Study in California.

4. When limiting beliefs or other risk factors are noted, therapy is indicated as soon as possible. Obstetrical histories should search for such conflict.

5. Decreasing maternal emotional and physical stress is important.

Passivity Vs. Activity

One last issue deserves mentioning—the difference between an active and passive attitude. In labor and preparing for labor, women need to be encouraged to remain active for as long as possible. Particularly for first labors, contractions are all consuming to a woman's attention. Having never had the experience before, many primagravidac mentally race ahead of their body process, expecting the baby to be born soon, when in actuality they are in early labor. The attitude of activity is emphasized by the realistic approach to childbirth as including a concept of *healthy* pain. The woman is directed to measure the progress of labor as relative to the quality of activity she is able to do in between contractions and not during the contraction itself. In this manner, a woman is encouraged to go about her daily activities (eating, sleeping, reading, baking, etc.) and to continue these activities throughout early labor, stopping only for contractions, but returning to her project when the contraction is over. The body leads a woman into hard labor, rather than the case of her mind jumping ahead of the process. The advantage is that a woman's behavior is influenced by an active approach to labor. If a woman takes a more passive approach, lying down in early labor, focusing on contractions, she is prone towards not sleeping and not eating. Simply waiting for the baby to be born in this manner can become quite exhaustive. Through an active approach, once again a woman is less likely to develop uterine intertia due to fatigue or having been awake for one or two nights, and having not eaten for 24 hours. The latter behavior is related to attitude. Childbirth classes should address attitude, thereby influencing behavior in favor of optimal mind-body integration for childbirth. The ability to work with pain in labor can be taught as an active approach which diminishes the possibility of becoming "victim" to the pain, and thereby alienated from the body. A response to pain by a "victim" attitude is a passive one, not conducive to normal delivery.

With the advantage of such preparation of this kind, women can be assessed on the basis of their attitudinal approach to life in general to determine possible delivery outcomes. Where a woman falls on, for example, the continuum of passivity vs. activity can already be assessed in her present lifestyle. Our belief is that a woman gives birth as she lives, the process of birth being secondary to and reflected in her manner of living. Effective preparation is seen as a possible change agent for developing coping skills within individual life styles, in which attitudes that may ill dispose a woman for coping with labor are changed or modified.

In this paper, prediction of outcome is based on our psychophysiological assessment after or towards the end of childbirth classes. Partially solidified change in beliefs and attitudes towards the end of classes may account for a certain amount of unpredictability and in part for the missed predictors in Table IX, Prediction Group 3.

REFERENCES

1. Simonton, O. C., Matthews-Simonton, S., and Creighton, T. *Getting Well Again*. Los Angeles: Tarcher Press, 1978.

2. Aubry, R. H. and Pennington, J. C. Identification and Evaluation of High-Risk Pregnancy: The Perinatal Concept. *Clin. Obstet. Gynecol.* 161 (1):3-27, March 1973.

3. Goodwin, J. E., Dunne, J. T., and Thomas B. W. Antepartum Identification of the Fetus at Risk. *Can. Med. Assoc. J.* 101:57, 1969.

4. Nesbitt, R. E., Jr. and Aubry, R. H. High-risk obstetrics II. Value of Semi-objective Grading System in Identifying the Vulnerable Groups. *Am. J. Obstet. Gynecol.* 103:972, 1969.

5. Hobel, C. J., Hyvarinen, M. A., Okada, D. M., and Oh, W. Prenatal and Intrapartum High-risk Screening. I. Prediction of high-risk neonate. *Am. J. Obstet. Gynecol.* 117:1, 1973.

6. Mondanlou, H., Yeh. S. Y., and Hon, E. H. Fetal and Neo-natal Acid-base Balance in Normal and High-risk Pregnancies During Labor and the First Hour of Life. *Obstet. Gynecol.* 43:347, 1974.

7. Yeh, S., Forsythe, A., Lowensohn, R. I., Hom, E. H. A Study of the Relationship Between Goodwin's High Risk Score and Fetal Outcome. *Am. J. Obstet. Gynecol.* 127 (1):50-55, 1977.

8. Butler, N. R. and Alderman. E. D. *Perinatal Problems: The Second Report of the 1958 British Perinatal Morality Survey.* Edinburgh: E. & S. Livingstone, Lt., 1969.

9. Shapiro, S., Schlesinger, E. R., Nesbitt, R. E. L., Jr. *Infant, Perinatal, Maternal and Childhood Mortality in the United States.* Cambridge, Mass.: Harvard Univ. Press, 1968, p. 1-388.

10. Ratakallio, P. Groups at Risk in Low-birth Weight Infants and Perinatal Morality. *Acta Paediatrica Scandinavica*, Supple. 193:5. 1969.

11. Glaser, B. *Theoretical Sensitivity: Advances in the Methodology of Grounded Theory.* Mill Valley: Sociology Press, 1978.

12. Koestenbaum, P. Phenomenological Foundations for the Behavioral Sciences: The Nature of the Facts. In: *The Vitality of Death.* Westport, Conn.: Greenwood Press, 1974.

13. Koestenbaum, P. Phenomenological Foundations for the Behavioral Sciences: The Method of Science. *Op. cit.*

14. Kosetenbaum, P. *Clinical Philosophy: The New Image of the Person.* Westport, Conn.: Greenwood Press, 1978.

15. Mehl, L. E., Peterson, G. H. Shaw, N., Crevy, D. Complications of Home Delivery. Analysis of a Series of 287 Deliveries From Santa Cruz, California *Birth and the Family Journal.* 2(4):123-131, 1975.

16. Mehl, L. E., Peterson, G. H., Whitt, M. and Hawes, W. Outcome of 1146 Elective Home Births. *J. Reproductive Med.* 19(3):281-290, 1977.

17. Peterson, G. H. and Mehl, L. E. Some Determinants of Maternal Attachment. *Am. J. Psychiat.* 135(10):1168-1173, 1978.

18. Peterson. G. H., Mehl, L. E., Lederman, P. H. Some Determinants of Father Attachment. *Am. J. Orthopsychiatry* 49(2):330-338, 1979.

19. Mehl, L. E., and Peterson, G. H. Berkeley Family Health Center. The Existential-phenomenological Approach to Holistic Health Care. In Stewart, D. and Stewart. L. *Freedom of Choice in Childbirth.* Marble Hill, MO: NAPSAC, 1979, Vol. II.

20. Mehl, L. E., et al. The Existential-phenomenological Approach to Childbirth: Needs Assessment. In: Stewart and Stewart, *op. cit.,* Vol. III.

21. Mehl, L. E. and Peterson, G. Existential Risk Screening. In Ahmed, P. (ed.) *Psychosocial Aspects of Pregnancy.* New York: Elsevier-North Holland, 1981.

22. Kerner, J. and Ferris, C. An Alternative Birth Center in a Community Teaching Hospital. *Ob Gyn.* 51(3):371-373, March 1978.

23. Mehl, L. E., and Peterson, G. H. *Holistic Prenatal Care,* Berkeley, Mindbody Press, in press.

Appendix One

Awareness Exercises

I. The Limbic System and Visualization

Many people may wonder how visualization can have an affect on physical manifestation. However, the fact that attitudes and emotional moods influence physical functioning in the body is not unknown. Popular belief in the mind as separate from the body has blinded many people to their interrelationship. It has already been mentioned that affective states or moods, such as depression, can affect the functioning of the immune system. However, the relevance of the limbic system to the visualization process deserves attention.

The hypothalamus releases hormones in the body and responds to emotional feelings in order to do so. In this way, one might think of the hypothalamus as the mediator of emotion, affecting physical functioning. As in the case of labor, the firing of oxytocin occurs in the posterior pituitary gland located in the hypothalamus, a part of the limbic system. In time of fright, the firing of oxytocin in labor is suppressed. This makes sense in line with the safeguards of nature. If a mother deer were giving birth and a lion approached, she would indeed need to stop her labor and run for safety. If her body did not respond to fright, her labor would continue in the midst of a life-threatening situation. Birth and death have their ways of sidestepping one another in such encounters. Likewise, anger has been found to often increase the firing of oxytocin from the posterior pituitary gland.

Sexual hormones are also released from the pituitary gland, and I have theorized, based on clinical experience, that some women have trouble with obtaining regular ovulation and are also in the midst of an identity crisis with regards to some aspect of womanhood. Psychotherapy around these issues may bring on regular ovulation if desired. Favorable results have been achieved in a like manner with habitual aborters desiring to be mothers.[1] Feelings are mediated through the limbic system and can affect physical functioning in the body.

The limbic system is connected to a secondary visual cortex through which, I hypothesize, visualization affects physical functioning. As the two visual cortices are paced together, an emotional experience results which may, with repeated focus, create a physical response, such as a hormonal release in the pituitary gland or the hypothalamus. One could further hypothesize that other neurochemical and neurohormonal effects may take place that are not yet measurable by modern science. The suggestion of such an occurrence may be interpreted from a study at Johns Hopkins University by John Tyler, et. al., involving the use of anesthetic cream on nursing mothers' nipples. Infants suckled their mothers' nipples, both with and without anesthetic cream on the nipples. With use of anesthetic cream, the mother was unable to feel the suckling to a large extent. Although mechanistically speaking, the infants' stimulus of sucking remained the same, the mother's inability to feel the actual suckling suppressed the "let down" response. This study suggests the presence of neurochemical or neurohormones that are not yet identified as playing an integral role in physical functioning. The ability to feel the experience of suckling also gives rise to emotional experience, as in childbirth, the ability to feel the process may contribute to an emotional experience, which is otherwise blocked. Blocking the ability to feel sensation in labor, breastfeeding, making love or other life processes, may also block the emotional response which can interfere with the release of neurochemicals or neurohormones needed to fulfill the physical process. The interrelationship of mind and body is more intricately and delicately entwined with emotions than has been appreciated by science in general.

The study of the body by the medical scientists and the study of the mind or the psyche by psychologists has contributed greatly to our exploration of how we work, how we are constructed as living people. However, the integral link between the two, the emotional reality of each and every experience as it occurs in our lives, is the manifestation of each discipline in the other. To deny the link any longer is not only impossible but disadvantageous to both the medical world and to psychology. Denial would constitute a blockage of further exploration of the study of the human being. We are able to study what makes up a liver, a heart, a brain, and the structure of each living cell in each organ. We are able to categorize, to label, to pronounce states of living matter. But we do not know how or why each cell exists as it does, why it lives, why it dies, how it got here. The living fetus throughout the 9 months of pregnancy can be understood as it progresses through developmental stages. It can be described. Each cell, each tissue that becomes is understood for its contents and relatively predictive progress. But how it can exist, be made from the depths of a woman's body, a man's sperm, on the outside of his physical self—the initiation and the secret of living matter and physical process remains unexplored by medical scientists.

Studying the emotional sphere and its interrelationship in life's manifestation of the human body will not give us all the answers. But it can begin the needed exploration of the meaning of emotional experience on the physical plane. Perhaps medical researchers have been studying the human body from a limited perspective of physical functioning to explain what life is. Now it is time to broaden medical minds with the study of emotional experience as it manifests itself on an intimately physical level.

II. Early Classes

During the course of development of prenatal classes, it became apparent that benefit could be derived from extending early classes from 2 classes to 3. In addition to the sensate focus exercise, which will be described shortly, the advantage of a prenatal thematic apperception test became apparent. The prenatal TAT is simply a series of cards, with images of pregnant women in different settings as well as pictures of newborns and male representations. Class members are asked to take copies of the cards home and to write descriptive stories describing each scene, which they can bring back to the next class to share with other members. Much insight and widening of horizons is possible with such an exercise. It has good results when given as homework in the second class, and brought back for discussion in the third class. Such an exercise facilitates opening the door to issues of deeper meaning involved in the roles of expectations of parenthood. Each individual is free to look inside themselves, to the depth that is comfortable for them. They may then choose further exploration if desirable, by the fact that such a perspective has been opened to them. The perspective of self-reflection itself may enrich the experience of the pregnancy and further heighten consciousness in parenting.

Sensate Focus

Sensate focus is an exercise used as homework between the first and second classes (or sometimes may be interchanged with the TAT and given between the second and third classes). It is an exercise initially developed by Masters and Johnson to enable couples to explore sensuality and sexuality outside of a framework of performance on a sexual level. The following instructions are given:

"In the next week, set aside some time alone together to explore one another's body. The agreement should be that this activity is not to culminate in sexual intercourse, and for this first time the genitals and breasts shall be considered off limits. Let the man begin by lying down first on his back, letting the woman begin at his head, caressing, exploring with hand and/or lips the front part of his body down to his toes (genitals excluded). Then he may turn on his stomach, so that she may continue to caress and explore his body from this perspective. This exercise may also be done taking turns, with each of you facing the other, sitting in a cross-legged position. Done in either position, both partners should take turns caressing and being caressed. The person being caressed should totally focus on what it feels like to be touched in this manner, also bringing his/her attention to the feeling such touching evokes in various parts of the body. The person touching should be focused on the sensation of touch and exploration. Eyes may be closed if desired, so as to increase the focus on sense of touch. Do not talk during the first time you do the exercise, just experience, afterwards sharing the experience with one another verbally, describing what you liked about the experience, what you didn't like, what it felt like in general.

Remember that it is imperative that you do not engage in sexual intercourse during or following this exercise, as it is one in which exploration of sensation and feeling is fully explored out of the context of any goal orientation or anxiety concerning performance in sex."

Couples are then able to come back and discuss what feelings, sensations, or issues were brought up around this exercise. It is an opening for exploring sexual issues as they arise in pregnancy. Many people may benefit simply from hearing others express their own experiences.

With the use of the prenatal TAT and the sensate focus exercise, couples are not necessarily involved in a lengthy psychological endeavor, but rather they are simply introduced to some psychosexual aspects of pregnancy. This introduction can serve to lessen inhibitions during labor and to enrich their own experience of pregnancy, birth, and parenthood.

III. Deep Breathing for Pushing in Second Stage of Labor

During the course of teaching breathing exercises, it became necessary to further exemplify the nature of breathing for pushing in second stage. As I teach that second stage is a natural progression of labor (and not an isolation, separated by an island called "transition") breathing for second stage is also a natural deepening of the breath, as a woman bears down to help push the baby out. Demonstration of this kind of deepening of breath out is by far the most advantageous method for teaching it. However the following instructions may describe this process:

First stage breathing: "Breathe in deeply through your nose, letting the breath out with a gentle hissing sound from the mouth, so that you can feel the air passageway as the breath comes out through the body. Feel the collapse of the lungs, the air passageway, as the breath comes out, relaxing down into your body as you do so." (Demonstration and practice follows.)

Second stage breathing: "Now, as the baby continues to make its passage down the birth canal, your breathing will follow. At this point, sound may also be elicited if it hasn't been already. The difference is that the exhale will be continued far deeper into the diaphragm and through to the psoas muscle, helping to form a muscular wall from which to push the baby downwards. At this point, sound may increase the strength and resistance of this muscular wall, which may be thought of as helping the baby in much the same way that a swimmer might use the cement wall of the swimming pool to push off from with his/her feet in order to propel themselves further out into the pool.

"Follow your breath out in the same manner in which you did with the earlier breathing, only this time, when you get to the bottom or end of the breath where it ends naturally, assume there is more air in the bottom and you need to push it out. As you do this, you will notice how the abdomen comes into play and how the pelvis tips upwards a bit." There should be a ripple of the pelvic and abdominal muscles (as well as the diaphragm and psoas muscle deep in the inside) all working together in a *sequential* progressive thrust outwards through the vagina. Demonstration follows in both a sitting position with legs crossed and lying down flat on the back to further illustrate the thrust of the pelvis.

Using the hissing sound out through the mouth on the exhale is important here as the point at which the pushing occurs can actually be heard. The point at which the earlier deep breathing would end should sound as natural as the end of a sigh. Where the exhale continues then sounds like a surge of air being further compressed out of a balloon which has already been half emptied through a small hole at the bottom.

Attention is called to the physical posture taken on during this kind of deeper breathing for activating the pelvic muscles. As the air is further pushed out on the exhale, the same posture is experienced as that of orgasm. This is especially notable in the demonstration if the teacher is lying flat on her back on the floor. The link between sexual orgasm and birth is also obvious during this exercise. Labor and birth are part of the sexual cycle, involving deep pelvic contractions as is true in the state of orgasm. Demonstration and practice takes place until everyone possesses an understanding of the importance of the breath out, which deepens in pushing.

In teaching breathing, the focus on the exhale is as important as the focus on the inhale. Too often, childbirth teachers emphasize the depth of the inhale and do not teach a complete exhale. When this happens, there is a tendency to hold onto the breath which may inhibit the effectiveness of pushing. After a complete inhale the emphasis of the exhale is significant, as the focus of the body in second stage will be to push out the baby, just as the breath is also being pushed out of the body.

If the second stage breathing is done as instructed, the activity of the pelvis is natural and is a secondary response to the motivation to push the rest of the air out of the body.

REFERENCES

1. Gadpaille, W. *Cycles of Sex*. New York, Charles Scribner and Sons, 1975.

Appendix Two

Breastfeeding and Nutrition

Pam England, C.N.M. and Lyn Jones

Breastfeeding provides an opportunity for emotional bonding between mother and child as well as optimal newborn nutrition and increased immunitiy against many diseases[1–13,31].

The breast produces milk on a supply and demand basis*. When the baby sucks on the breast, the milk storage sinuses are compressed and milk flows through the nipple. The more frequently the baby nurses, the greater the milk supply. A message is sent via the nervous system to the hypothalamus of the brain and then to the pituitary gland. The pituitary gland responds by producing the hormones of prolactin, responsible for stimulating milk production in the breast, and oxytocin, which helps to release milk from the production cells into the storage ducts[14–17]. The "let-down reflex" refers to the release of milk from the alveoli, or storage areas of the breast, into the ducts leading to the nipple. A sensation of increased pressure in the breast is usually associated with this let-down[14,18–21]. Certain substances in high enough concentrations may inhibit the let-down among some women, including caffeine, (found in coffee, tea, chocolate, and soft drinks), some other drugs, including cigarettes (particularly over ten per day), labor medications or maternal illness[14]. Other drugs may also affect the ease of let-down, and substances such as alcohol and B-vitamins may help to promote the let-down for other women; hence, the advice given to some new mothers to drink dark, rich in yeast, imported beer when let-down is being inhibited.

---

*The breast consists of two major compartments. The first, primarily responsible for milk production, consists of an accumulation of alveoli, or specialized milk production cells, that discharge milk into conducting channels known as lactiferous ducts. The ends of these passageways dilate to store the milk and are located under the areola (the brownish area around the nipple). These storage areas are called lactiferous sinuses[14].

While newly breastfeeding women are often told to "Relax and be well rested!," in order to breastfeed, most women do experience tension and interrupted sleep during the postpartum period and yet are still able to breastfeed. While rest and relaxation is optimal for breastfeeding, it is certainly not a requirement.

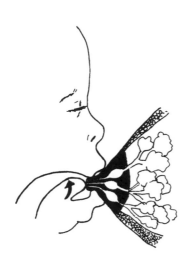

If the baby's gums press on or just behind the nipple, milk cannot be released from the sinuses and the nipple will become sore.

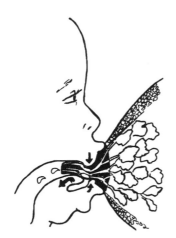

In order to breastfeed, a baby must squeeze milk from the sinuses beneath the areola into the nipple by pressing its jaws against the areola. The nipple is then drawn into the mouth and against the palate by the foreward, upward and backward motion of the tongue and sucking. When the mouth fills with milk, the baby swallows which is another way of knowing the baby is nursing correctly.

Common Questions About Breastfeeding

1. *How long? How often?*

Normal, healthy babies thrive on nursing from 10 to 60 minutes in duration at each feeding. Some babies need to suck longer than others to feel satisfied. Unlimited nursings are important in establishing an adequate supply of milk. Problems with nipple damage rarely occur from unrestricted nursing *if* the baby is positioned properly at the breast. Nursing limited to 5 minutes at a feeding often only serve to inhibit let-down reflex with associated frustration for some babies who do not receive enough milk to satisfy them.

Nursing patterns will change as the baby grows, and during illness or periods of emotional upsets. Nursing on demand seems optimal for the gestalt of mother and baby.

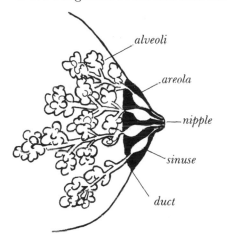

Often women are told that the baby obtains most of the milk in the first 10 minutes of sucking and that sucking thereafter is recreational, implying that it is probably unnecessary, or that enjoyment at the breast is improper and/or frivolous in our work-ethic society. Many let-down's may actually occur during each nursing, even if the mother usually feels only one. The breast may continue to produce milk in response to the suck even after 10 or 20 minutes. As milk is drained from the storage sinuses underneath the areola, the alveoli are continually adding milk to those storage areas. It does not totally empty, and therefore, may not require a period of "rest" in order to "rebuild the milk supply," as some authorities indicate.

While there are similarities among nursing babies' schedules, their patterns cannot be compared too closely. For example, such patterns may continue or change often unpredictably, yet remain normal. While some babies nurse vigorously immediately after birth, others seem tired and show little interest in nursing for several hours. Both responses are normal.

Most nursing infants need to nurse every 1 1/2 to 3 hours during the day, since breast milk lactalbumin protein is easily digested. Formula is digested more slowly and has more tryptophan and less zinc, magnesium and trace metals than human milk, perhaps providing a partial explanation for the formula-fed baby's sometimes sleeping longer between feedings and awakening with more irritability.*

2. *What about growth spurts?*

Periodically, babies go through growth spurts and want to nurse more often for 24 to 48 hours. If the baby is allowed to nurse on demand through these important days, more milk will be produced and the baby's appetite can be satisfied. Growth spurts commonly occur around the 7–10th day, 2 weeks, 4–6 weeks and again at 6 months. Babies, however, may not have learned these important dates and may differ a great deal from schedule.

3. *How do you know when a baby is getting enough milk?*

When a baby is gaining weight at a rate of 1/2 to 1 1/2 ounces per day (after the usual weight loss of up to 10% of its birth weight during the first week after birth), wetting 6–8 diapers per day and nursing 6–12 times a day, that baby is certainly receiving enough milk. Some of the possible indications that a baby is not getting enough are weight loss, poor weight gain and/or a seeming dissatisfaction represented by the baby nursing constantly. Consultation with a breastfeeding counselor might be a valuable resource if these events occur.

In addition, infants usually double their birth weight by 6 months and triple it by one year. Their length is usually 1 1/2 times their birth length at one year and the head circumference

---

*One study from the John Radcliffe Hospital in Oxford, England, found that infants allowed unlimited access to the breast actually fed less often than babies placed upon a clock schedule during their first two days of life. At the end of one week, both groups fed about the same number of times per day[22].

usually grows 3 inches. If such growth does not occur, an individual assessment is recommended.

4. *What can be done if the baby is not getting enough milk?*

Virtually all women are capable of breastfeeding, including women who have not given birth, but have adopted babies,[26] women who have weaned and wish to resume nursing,[24] and even insulin-dependent diabetic mothers. Many problems that do arise are related to the baby's suck, and not the woman's breast. Babies can learn improper sucking patterns shortly after birth. An immature nervous system, drugs given during labor or birth, early bottles, or too long an interval between birth and the baby's first nursing are often related to such learning. Sucking problems may be suspected in the presence of a discontented baby, with or without poor weight gain, mastitis (breast infection) developing early postpartum or constantly sore or cracked nipples.

With patience and help, a baby can be taught to suck properly. The situation is complicated if bottle feeding is introduced to supplement feeding as it can foster nipple confusion and decrease the supply of breast milk[27]. If the baby needs additional calories, an eye dropper, spoon or a Lact-aid* can be used instead of a supplemental bottle[24,34].

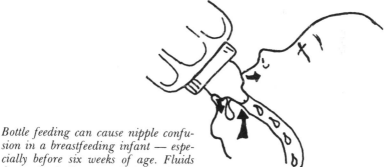

Bottle feeding can cause nipple confusion in a breastfeeding infant — especially before six weeks of age. Fluids from a bottle flow so easily into a baby's mouth, the vigorous sucking and the jaw and tongue motions necessary to breast feed are not needed. In fact, babies may need to curl their tongues forward and over the bottle's nipple to slow down the flow. Thus, teaching the baby incorrect sucking pattern and confusion at the breast.

5. *How can sore nipples be prevented?*

Many childbirth educators have instructed women to "toughen" their nipples in preparation for the baby's strong suck, with nipple rolling, exposure to the sun and gently rubbing with a washcloth being the most commonly recommended methods. Such practices may or may not be helpful, but are not harmful. However, a woman who has painstakenly prepared her nipples steadfastly believing she will have no soreness, only to experience soreness when the baby latches on, may feel confused. Some studies have shown that women who "prepare" have no less nipple soreness than women who do not. However, if a woman is familiar with touching, seeing or exposing her breasts, emotional preparation through physical manipulation prenatally may facilitate comfort and lack of inhibition for breastfeeding. The woman with flat or inverted nipples will be saved needless anxiety and difficulty if educated and prepared prenatally. The true inverted nipple retracts when pinched, instead of protruding. This is fairly uncommon. More commonly, the flat nipple, when pinched, will not invert or retract, but won't protrude very much[24]. Both problems can be treated with a plastic breast cup or shield worn during pregnancy. The shield helps break down the adhesions around the nipple, thus allowing the nipple to protrude so as to be more easily accessible to the baby. The hard plastic "cup" breast shields (see drawing) should not be confused with the pliable nipple shields which are not helpful.

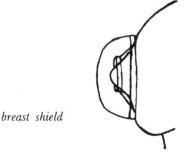

breast shield

Positioning for Breastfeeding

One aid to decreasing nipple soreness is the optimal positioning of the baby at the breast, along with nursing on demand (unlimited access to the breast and unlimited lengths of feeds).

The drawings illustrate the guidelines for one common and useful position:

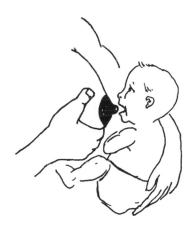

proper position

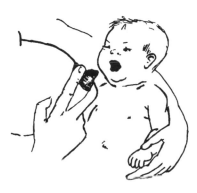

improper position

If the baby is not held close enough, the baby may grasp the nipple only, instead of the areola and nipple. This will cause soreness and may not allow enough stimulation to provide baby with adequate milk.

1. Place the baby's head in the crook of arm. This frees the opposite hand to hold baby's bottom or legs.
2. The baby's tummy and hips will face the mother's abdomen.
3. Support the mother's arm with pillows.
4. With the opposite hand, cup or hold the breast between the thumb and fingers.
5. Tickle baby's mouth with the nipple — when baby's mouth is open wide, bring *baby to the nipple.* mouth should cover as much of the areola as possible (it will not be all covered on a large areola). The areola is the darker colored part of the breast which includes, but is not limited to the nipple itself.
6. If the baby feels off-centered on the areola or has not taken in enough of the areola, gently insert a finger in the corner of baby's mouth and press against the breast to break the suction and begin again.

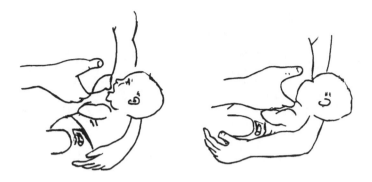

As previously mentioned, optimal positioning of the baby at the breast and unlimited access to the breast have been the best insurance against sore nipples in our clinical practice. In addition, in our practice we make the following recommendations:

1. Moderate use of lanolin, vitamin E oil or vegetable oil applied to the nipple after feedings. Do not use breast creams with directions to wash off before nursing as natural emoillents excreted by the nipple will also be washed away.
2. Expose nipples to air between nursings. Prolonged wearing of breast pads fosters sore nipples and may encourage growth of bacteria or monilia (a yeast infection).
3. Allow baby to nurse both breasts each feeding, beginning with the side which is least sore so that the initial vigorous sucking does not aggravate the sore nipple.
4. Apply ice to the nipples before the baby latches on.
5. Do not wash with soap which tends to dry the nipples.
6. Five to ten minutes of direct sunlight per day or heat from a lamp.
7. If the nipples are so sore that a long feeding is extremely painful, a woman can limit the feeding to 5 minutes per breast if she switches breasts several times during the nursing so that each breast is adequately emptied and the baby is certain to obtain enough milk.

Breast Engorgement

Breast engorgement may develop during the first week post partum, related to an increased blood flow to the breasts[32] and from a stasis of milk in the breast, sometimes in association with limited or scheduled nursings or an infant with a poor suck. The mother's temperature may be slightly elevated and the breasts may be swollen. Tender and small lumps are often felt. Prevention or cure of engorgement is usually accomplished with unlimited nursing every 2–3 hours and warm, moist heat, showers, or ice packs. At most, the problem will usually resolve in several days.

Breast Infection or Plugged Ducts

Breast infection (mastitis) or plugged ducts sometimes occur during the first few months post partum. Usually one breast is affected with a red, tender area, hot to the touch and one or several lumps can be felt. The woman may have a fever of 103° or 104°F and feel general achiness, nausea, loss of appetite and lethargy.

If conservative treatment is begun early, the infection will usually subside in 24 hours. A common treatment regimen is the following: apply warm, moist compresses to the affected breast, take a hot shower or bath at least 10 to 20 minutes every 3–4 hours; drink plenty of fluids and go to bed to rest, nursing the baby no less that every 2–3 hours beginning each on the affected breast to insure complete emptying[29]. Asking a friend or relative to assist with meals and household responsibilities during this 24 hour period so the woman can be on bed rest may be important as well.

Plugged ducts and breast infections are very similar in symptoms and treatment. Both may relate to prolonged periods between nursings (more than 3–4 hours), incomplete emptying of the breasts in association with limited nursing or poor sucking patterns of the baby, improper positioning, cracked nipples, wearing too tight a bra, or in an over-active, over-tired mother.

If the fever or symptoms are still present after 24 hours, a midwife or physician should be consulted. Rarely, a breast infection will progress to an abcess which requires antibiotics and may need to be surgically drained of the pus in a clinic or hospital[30]. It is important for the mother to continue nursing even if this should occur.

Cesareans and Breastfeeding

After a cesarean, the side lying position is usually most comfortable for breastfeeding. Pillows placed under the abdomen to prevent sagging and pulling on the incision and a rolled blanket or small pillow between the abdomen and the baby to prevent the baby from kicking the incision can be helpful.

If the mother nurses sitting up, it is helpful to place a pillow under the knees in bed, or a foot stool under the feet if in a chair, to reduce strain on the incision and again, a pillow over the abdomen.

If any of the following problems are encountered, additional help may be necessary:

1. Persistent sore nipples;
2. cracked nipples (visible fissures on nipple itself);
3. plugged ducts or mastitis (localized, red, tender, swollen areas of a breast);
4. a baby who sleeps constantly and is difficult to arouse;
5. a baby who is not producing 6–8 very wet diapers per 24 hours;
6. a baby who is losing weight after the first two weeks, or who had not regained his/her birthweight by 3 weeks;
7. a baby who seems constantly discontent and who wants to suck *all* of the time (hours at a time) and fusses as soon as he/she is put down.

Nutrition and Breastfeeding

In pregnancy some of the weight gained is stored in fat cells throughout the body. When nursing begins, some of the calories needed for making milk are supplied through the mobilization of this fat from storage to milk production. The amount of milk produced varies in relation to the quality of the woman's diet and the length of time she has been nursing. If her diet is calorie deficient, she may make less milk. A nursing woman's caloric needs also vary in relation to her weight gain during pregnancy, her activity and how long she has been nursing.

A non-pregnant woman usually requires an average of 2000 calories per day to maintain a stable weight. A nursing women usually needs an additional 900 calories a day. During the first few months of nursing, her body mobilizes some of the fat stores laid down during pregnancy to supply a third of these caloric needs. The other 500 calories are be provided from the diet. (Refer to Table 1 – Diet.)

At a certain time, which differs from woman to woman but

often occurs around three months postpartum, her body will have used up these fat stores. This is also a time when some women have relaxed the quality of their diet. It is important to continue to be aware of the growing baby's needs and increase caloric intake an extra 400 calories to meet the 2900 calories a day usually required. If a substantial weight gain, (35–40 pounds) occurred during pregnancy, the woman's fat stores will probably last longer than three months. If she is very active or athletic, she may need to increase her calories accordingly. Eating an adequate diet without the need for excessive rapid weight reduction is useful for maintaining an adequate milk supply. This is not a good time to fast or to reduce weight rapidly.

For nursing twins, approximately 4000 calories and 80–100 grams of protein a day are usually needed. (The No-Risk diet plus 2 cups of milk – Table 1.) It is important for the pregnant woman expecting twins to eat at least 3100 calories and 110–130 grams of protein daily to expect a weight gain of approximately 40 or more pounds. An adequate diet facilitates term pregnancy and the ability to nurse afterwards.

Protein and Calcium

The amount of protein in a diet determines the amount of calcium needed. Too little protein can result in decreased calcium absorption while an excessive amount of protein may increase calcium loss through the urine. The usual recommended daily allowance for non-pregnant women is 44 grams of protein and 500mg (0.5 gram) of calcium per day. Because many Americans consume more than the RDA* for protein, calcium requirements for pregnancy have been written as 800mg a day. Nursing women generally require 65–75 grams of protein and 1200mg of calcium daily. (See Table 1.)

Protein and calcium levels in breast milk remain relatively constant regardless of dietary intake, these substances being mobilized from body stores if not present in the diet. If the diet is sufficiently calcium deficient during breastfeeding, the bones can lose calcium at a rate of up to 250mg per day (the amount secreted in breast milk per day) to provide calcium to the baby. Such calcium loss, if very extreme could become a precursor to the development of osteoporosis*. It is preferable and easy to provide adequate calcium through the diet.

---

*RDA (Recommended Daily Allowance)
*Osteoporosis is a condition consisting of calcium loss from the bones with the bones becoming brittle to the point of breaking easily.

Alternatives to Milk/Dairy

4 cups of milk daily or foods equivalent to 1200mg calcium are needed to supply adequate calcium. 1 cup of milk equals 300mg of calcium. Other choices equal to a cup of milk are:*

1 cup yogurt
1 1/2 oz natural cheese
1 1/3 cup cottage cheese
1 1/2 cup natural ice cream
2/3 cup sardines
1 cup almonds
2 cups sesame seeds
1 1/2 cup tahini
2 tbsp Blackstrap molasses
1/2 cup carob flour/powder
2 tbsp kelp
6 cups soymilk (not calcium fortified)
2 cups soybeans (not calcium fortified)
1/2 lb tofu
2 cups cooked broccoli
1 cup mustard greens
1 cup turnip greens
2 cups cooked dandelion greens
1 cup collard greens
1 cup Hijiki
1 cup wakame

Calcium absorption is improved in the presence of fat. Eating some fat-containing foods (cheese, mayonnaise, meat, salad oil, etc.) at the same time as eating calcium-containing foods will actually increase the percent absorption of calcium. Chocolate decreases calcium absorption binding with the calcium to form an unusable product. If drinking 3-4 glasses of milk a day is difficult, creamed soups, cheese sauces on vegetables, and yogurt substituted for mayonnaise or cream in sauces, dips and salad dressing may be considered. Alternately a protein drink or calcium supplements may provide the needed calcium and are

---

*Note: Fast food "shakes," malts, soft ice cream do not contain real milk but are chemical imitations. Bancha tea, sometimes recommended as a calcium source, may be unreliable. Rebecca Greenwood, of the East West Foundation in Boulder, reports that her sources indicate that a cup of brewed, bancha twig tea contains 7.2mg of calcium. A chemical analysis by *Celestial Seasonings* revealed that brewed bancha tea contains caffeine and tannin. Tannin can impede iron absorption.

sometimes very helpful when nutritional deficiencies have been long standing. A recipe for one is included after Table 1.

What About Vitamin Supplements?

Vitamin supplements are not a substitute for good eating. Vitamins are preferable taken in their natural food sources. Vitamins taken during pregnancy can often be continued into nursing. Consultation with a holistic health practitioner might help in terms of adjusting vitamin intake to complement diet and possible deficiencies and needs. Vitamins are generally not harmful except for some taken in megadoses.

Body stores of vitamins A, E, D, K, and some B vitamins may be depleted during nursing if intake is inadequate. Dr. Donsbach's Prenatal Formula is a good general vitamin found in health food stores for those women who do not have the knowledge of or access to holistic health care to individualize vitamin needs and dosages. If this is not available, average doses are vitamin A, 10,000 I.U.; vitamin E, 200 I.U.; folic acid, 800mcg; calcium, 750mg; iron, 20mg.

If body iron stores were depleted during pregnancy or more than the normal amount of blood was lost during childbirth, supplemental iron may be needed. Anemia is determined by a simple blood test (Hematocrit: the percentage of whole blood that is red blood cells) that can be done one week after birth. Some women have improved their body iron levels by adding foods high in iron and vitamin C sources to the diet. Some iron rich foods are meat and (organic) liver, brewer's yeast, molasses, apricots, raisins, prunes, whole grains, beans and green vegetables. Many nutrients, not just iron, help prevent and resolve anemia. An iron rich diet may still be inadequate if other deficiencies are present. Vitamin C, folic acid, B12, B6, calcium, copper and sufficient hydrochloric acid in the stomach are also needed to effectively assimilate iron.

If the anemia is severe or doesn't improve with iron rich foods by six weeks postpartum, a woman may need to supplement with amino acid-chelated iron and vitamin C in the doses recommended by the woman's health pracitioner or dictated by her own body awareness. Chelated iron is iron bound to protein molecules so as to pass more easily through the intestines into the blood. More iron is absorbed with less toxicity with chelated iron than with iron salts (ferrous sulfate and ferrous gluconate).

Zinc deficiency is also occasionally found in nursing mothers.

The 1980 Recommended Daily Allowance of zinc is 25mg per day. It is sometimes difficult to obtain this amount from food or average multi-vitamin-mineral supplements. When this occurs, zinc supplementation might be considered.

If supplemental calcium is needed, amino acid-chelated calcium is recommended. Dolomite is more difficult to absorb and sometimes contains toxic metals such as lead, arsenic, mercury and aluminum. Women may also keep in mind that life stress affects the body's ability to absorb vitamins and that continued deficiencies in the presence of adequate nutrition may indicate the need for stress reduction or family stress management. Counselling and therapy services can be utilized during postpartum family adjustment to decrease overall tension and may prove very beneficial in increasing milk supply in some instances, as well.

Do Babies Need Supplements?

The first six months, the baby does not need anything besides breast milk[33]. The best way to insure the baby's nutritional needs are being met has already been discussed for the mother to maintain her own adequate nutrition. Nursing the baby is the best thing to do nutritionally (as well as emotionally). Even if the woman thinks her diet is not as good as it should be, no formula will be better for her baby than her own breast milk.

Infant Anemia

First, the woman or her health practitioner may consider what is "anemic." Often this definition varies considerably. Paavo Airola, author of *Everywoman's Book,* states that anywhere from 9.8 to 12.6 grams of hemoglobin (the iron-containing portion of red blood cells) in the blood is considered normal for infants. In high altitudes a hemoglobin of 12gm% is normal at 2 months and 11gm% at 12 months with hematocrit levels from 35 to 38. Some causes listed by Airola for anemia in babies include:

1. insufficient storage supply of iron received at birth related to a deficient diet of the mother during pregnancy,
2. cutting of the umbilical cord before transfer of placental blood to the infant,
3. a severely deficient maternal diet during breastfeeding,
4. artificial formula feeding,

5. the baby's poor assimilation of iron and other blood building nutrients,
6. other health disorders that interfere with normal blood building process.

Premature babies or babies who had blood transfusions at birth are also more susceptible to anemia.

Iron in fortified formula and cereal is not easily absorbed. Breast milk has a constant trace of iron, even when the diet fluctuates from day to day. That iron is in a form most easily absorbed by the baby.

The amount of vitamins in the breast milk is largely dependent on the mother's dietary intake of vitamins and to a lesser degree on vitamin supplementation. Water soluble vitamins (B's and C's) are especially dependent on food intake, but fat soluble vitamin A seems to work this way also.

Recent research indicates that women who eat a diet of supplemented foods have higher vitamin contents in their milk than women who simply take vitamin supplements. It seems reasonable to conclude that eating whole, real foods are essential to maintaining the quantity and quality of milk needed by a growing baby.

Drugs and Breastfeeding

Generally speaking, many authorities argue that the need for the mother to take medications does not necessitate cessation of nursing. Doctors often choose particular medications from habit rather than a unique requirement for that particular drug. An "activated" client can assertively address this issue with the doctor, and doctor and client can then work together to choose a medication regimen safest for breastfeeding.

Erickson, et. al.[34] describe how mothers on tricyclic antidepressant drugs for postpartum depression need not discontinue nursing. They determine that the infant would only receive 0.04 mg/kg of antidepressant per day with the mother on therapeutic blood levels. The beginning therapeutic dosage for six year old children is 1mg/kg/day. As they state, "Given the desirability of breastfeeding for the infant and for the mother with depression and the extremely low concentrations of [the drug] likely to be present in breast milk, it seems unwarranted to recommend categorically that a nursing woman taking those drugs discontinue breastfeeding."[35] Such findings apply to many other drugs, as well. Information on other drugs is available[35–36].

Table 1 *PREGNANCY AND LACTATION NO RISK FOOD GUIDE*
each food may be counted for one group only
(except calcium group for vegans)

	Group I Eggs	Group II Dairy	Group III Vegetarian Protein Sources	Group IV Grain Products
Non-Vegetarian	2 servings	4 servings	as desired (can substitute for meat servings)	5 servings
Lacto-Ovo Vegetarian	2 servings	4 servings	3 servings	3 slices yeast raised whole grain bread and 2 other choices
Vegan* may need to supplement with calcium, B12	none	4 choices from Alternatives to Milk/Dairy	6 servings	5 slices yeasted bread and 4 other choices

	Group I Eggs	Group II Dairy	Group III Vegetarian Protein Sources	Group IV Grain Products
One Serving Equivalents	1 egg	1 C whole milk, buttermilk, yogurt, sour cream; 1/3 C powdered milk, 1¼ oz. hard cheese; 1¼ C cottage cheese.	(raw measures) 7 oz. tofu; 4 oz. tempeh; 2 c soy milk, ½ c peanuts or peanut butter; ¼ c beans + ½ c rice or wheat; ¼ c brewer's yeast + ½ c rice; ¼ c sesame or sunflower seeds + 1 c rice; ½ c rice + ⅔ c milk; 1 oz. cheese + 4 slices whole wheat bread or ⅔ c macaroni or noodles or ¼ c beans; ¼ c beans + 1 c cornmeal; ¼ c beans + ⅓ c seeds' ¼ c peanut butter or peanuts + ¼ c seeds; ½ c milk + ½ cup seeds; 1 lg potato + ½ c milk or ½ oz. cheese; 2 oz. hard cheese; ½ c cottage cheese	1 slice yeasted whole grain bread; 1 corn tortilla; ½ roll, bagel or muffin, 1 wholegrain waffle or pancake; ½ c hot cereal, rolled oats, cracked wheat; ¼ c wheat germ; ½ c cold cereal, granola; ½ c macaroni, noodles; ½ c cooked rice, millet, bulgur

* 1 serving of tempeh per week provides all the B12 needed.

While lactating, add 400 calories per day (2 cups of milk, 1/2 cup nuts or 2 servings grains) if the woman has returned to her pre-pregnant weight.

For lactation, less protein is required, but calories need to be maintained. One could delete 1–2 protein servings per day and add 2–3 grain servings.

Vegetarian information adapted from *Vegetarian Baby* by Yntema; non-vegetarian information is from the Society for the Protection of the Unborn through Nutrition (SPUN), which unfortunately no longer exists.

Group V Dark green vegetables	Group VI Fruits, vegetables rich in vitamin C	Group VII other fruits and vegetables	Group VIII Fats (oil)	Group IX Meat, poultry and fish
2 servings	2 servings	1 yellow fruit or vegetable	3 servings	4 servings
2 servings	2 servings	1 yellow fruit or vegetable	3 servings	none
3 servings	2 servings	2 yellow fruits or vegetables	4 servings	none

Group V Dark green vegetables	Group VI Fruits, vegetables rich in vitamin C	Group VII other fruits and vegetables	Group VIII Fats (oil)	Group IX Meat, poultry and fish
(raw measures) 1 c spinach; collards, mustard, dandelion; broccoli, kale; cabbage; asparagus; dark green lettuce or sprouts	1 orange or grapefruit; 4 oz. grapefruit juice, ½ cantaloupe; 1 lg tomato; ¾ c papaya or strawberries; 12 oz. tomato or pineapple juice; 2 lemons or limes, ¼ c green or red peppers	3 apricots; ½ cantaloupe; ½ c carrots, winter squash, pumpkin, 1 sweet potato	1 T butter, mayonnaise or vegetable oil, ¼ avocado, 1 T peanut butter	2 oz. chicken, beef, poultry, veal, liver, kidney, fish, ½ c canned tuna, salmon, mackerel, 6 sardines

Protein Calcium Drink

    2 tbsp powdered milk (whole, non-instant)
    2 tbsp peanut butter
    2 tbsp blackstrap molasses
    1 tbsp powdered carob
    1 egg
    1 tray ice cubes (if using food processor) or,
    1/2 tray ice cubes and 1 cup water or milk (if using blender)
    Put all ingredients together and blend until creamy. For more calcium and protein milk can be frozen in the ice trays. Makes two cups. Two cups of this drink will provide the following nutrients: calcium 526mgs, protein 18.6 grams, calories 425.

Sea Vegetables

Seaweed is an excellent source of calcium, vitamin A, and other vitamins and minerals. It may, however, be difficult to eat in large quantities. The taste of seaweed is strong and the method of preparation can help tremendously in its palatability. One suggestion is: soak seaweed until soft, and expanded in size. Rinse very well in clear water to get rid of the grittiness. Season with tamari and steam with thinly sliced carrots for 30 minutes.

REFERENCES

1. Pittard, W. B., "Special Properties of Human Milk," *Birth* 8(4): 229–243, 1981.

2. Bloom, M., "The Romance and Power of Breastfeeding," *Birth* 8(4): 259–269, 1981.

3. Fredrikzon, B., Hernell, O., Blackberg, L. and Olivecrona, T., "Bile Salt-Stimulated Lipase in Human Milk: Evidence of Activity *In Vivo* and of a Role in the Digestion of Milk Retinal Esters. *Pediat. Res.* 12:1048–1052, 1978.

4. Butler, J. E., "Immunological Aspects of Breastfeeding, Anti-Infectious Activity of Breast Milk." *Seminars in Perinatology* 3:255, July 1979.

5. Oseid, B., "Breastfeeding and Infant Health." *Seminars in Perinatology* 249–254, op. cit.

6. Jenness, R., "The Composition of Human Milk," *Seminars in Perinatology* 225, op. cit.

7. Nelson, B., "Breastfeeding Urged to Protect Teeth," *Los Angeles Times,* Wed., Oct. 29, 1975, p. 21.

8. Newton, N. and Newton, M., "Psychologic Aspects of Lactation," *New England Journal of Medicine* 277:1179–1188, 1967.

9. Eckhart, C. D., Sloan, M. V., Duncan, J. R., Hurley, L. G., "Zinc Binding: A Difference Between Human and Bovine Milk," *Science* 195:789–790, 1977.

10. Larsen, S. A. and Homer, D. R., "Relation of Breast Versus Bottle Feeding to Hospitalization for Gastroenteritis in a Middle-Class U.S. Population," *Journal of Pediatrics* 92(3):417–418, March 1978.

11. Jelliffe, D. B. and Patrice, Jelliffe, E. F., "Nutrition and Human Milk," *PostGraduate Medicine* 60(1):153–156, July 1976. 1976.

12. Hall, B., "Changing Composition of Human Milk and Early Development of an Appetite Control," *The Lancet,* 779–782 April 5, 1975.

13. Ounsted, M. and Sleigh, G., "The Infant's Self-Regulation of Food Intake and Weight Gain," *The Lancet,* 1393–1397, June 28, 1975.

14. Cerrutti, E. R., "The Management of Breastfeeding," *Birth* 8(4):251–265, 1981.

15. Applebaum, R. M., "The Modern Management of Successful Breastfeeding," *Pediat. Clin. No. Am.* 17:203, 1970.

16. Campbell, B., et. al., "Milk 'Let-Down' and the Orgasm in the Human Female," *Hum. Biol.* 25:165, 1953.

17. Cowie, A. T., "Overview of the Mammary Gland," J. *Invest. Derm.* 63:2, 1974.

18. Ely, F., et. al. "Factors Involved in the Ejection of the Milk," *Am. Jour. Dairy Sci.* 24:211, 1941.

19. Fowler, M., " A New Era in Breastfeeding," *J. Trop. Ped.* 22(2): 34, 1976.

20. Hytten, F. E., "The Physiology of Lactation," *J. Hum. Nutr.* 30:225, 1976.

21. Meites, J., "Neurophysiology of Lactation," *J. Invest. Derm.* 63:119, 1974.

22. "Demand in Feeding of Infant Won't Raise Frequency," *Family Practice News*, October 15, 1976, p. 12.

23. Newton, N., "Human Lactation," in Kon, S. K. and Cowie, A. T., *Milk: The Mammary Gland and Its Secretion*, New York: Academic Press, Vol. 1, 1961.

24. Waletzky, L. and Herman, E. C., "Relactation," *American Family Physician* 14(2):69–74, 1976.

25. Crozer-Griffith, J. P., "The Ability of Mothers to Nurse Their Children," *J. A. M. A.* 59:1874–1917, 1912.

26. Stein, R., "The Adoptive Mothers Who Breastfeed Their Tots," *San Francisco Chronicle* Tues., Nov. 27, 1973, p. 22.

27. Strom, J., "The Falling Rate of Breastfeeding in Sweden," *Acta. Paediat.* 45:453, 1956.

28. Miller, D. L., "Birth and Long-Term Unsupplemented Breastfeeding in 17 Insulin-Dependent Diabetic Mothers," *Birth* 4(2):65–70, 1977.

29. Marshall, B. R., Hiepper, J. K. and Zirbel, C. C., "Sporadic Puerperal Mastitis: An Infection That Need Not Interrupt Lactation," *J. A. M. A.* 233(13):1377–1380, 1975.

30. Smith, C. O. and Varga, A., "Puerperal Breast Abscess," *Am. J. Obst. and Gynec.* 74(6):1330–1341, 1957.

31. Brewster, D. P., *You Can Breastfeed Your Baby Even in Special Situations,* Rodale Press, Emmaus, PA, 1979.

32. Burd, L. I., Dorin, M., Philipose, V. and Lemons, J. A., "The Relationship of Mammary Temperature to Parturition in Human Subjects," *Amer. J. Obstet. and Gynec.* 128(3):272–278, 1977.

33. Smith, G. V., Calvert, L. J. and Kanto, W. P., "Breastfeeding and Infant Nutrition," *American Family Physician* 17(4):92–102, 1978.

34. Erickson, S. H., Smith, G. H. and Heidrick, F., "Tricyclics and Breastfeeding," *Am. J. Psychiatry* 136(11):1483, 1979.

35. Lipman, A. G., "Antimicrobials Excreted in Breast Milk," *Modern Medicine* March 15, 1977.

36. Lipman, A. G., "Drugs Excreted in Breast Milk," *Modern Medicine* 185–186, July 15–August 15, 1978.

ADDITIONAL RESOURCES

*Lact-aid, P. O. Box 1066, Atlens, TN 37303

LaLeche League International, 9616 Minneapolis Avenue, Franklin Park, IL 60131

Index